NOT ABOUT GOLF

NOT ABOUT GOLF

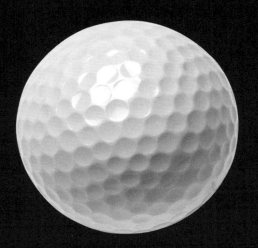

THE LIFE-CHANGING JOY
OF PLAYING THE GAME

ABOUT YOU & GOLF

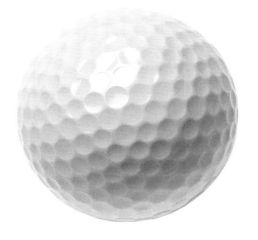

NATIONAL BESTSELLING AUTHOR
MIKE BERLAND

Regan Arts.

Regan Arts books may be purchased for
educational, business, or sales promotional use.
For information, please contact:
internationalrights@reganarts.com

First Regan Arts edition, June 2025
Library of Congress Control Number: 2024947543
ISBN: 978-1-68245-235-6 (eBook)
ISBN: 978-1-68245-234-9 (HC)

Design by Neuwirth & Associates, Inc.
Cover design by Maria Zarba and Matthew Werner

Printed in China
1   3   5   7   9   10   8   6   4   2

This book is dedicated to Greg
for introducing me to the game of golf.

It has had a life-changing impact on me,
my family, and my friends.

And to Shelly
for helping to keep me on course.

CONTENTS

SHARING GOLF'S SECRETS

When I sat down to write this book, my goal was to share the golf secrets that nobody talks about. I also wanted to debunk the myths and misconceptions that are perpetuated by those who don't understand or play golf but like to criticize it anyway. I'm not coming at this subject from the perspective of a golf professional. I'm not approaching it as a great player. (I didn't start golfing until I was twenty-one.) I'm not even an amazing amateur golfer. Nor do I work for a golf company or have any financial interest in golf. I am a pollster, a researcher, and an analyst who has worked for top corporations and political leaders. My job is to collect data, glean insights from the data, and offer advice and strategies. Whether that strategizing has been for Mike Bloomberg, Hillary Clinton, Airbnb, Facebook, Crocs, or the NHL, my clients have always counted on me to give them the straight facts and help them navigate the next steps.

I've had no such steady guide when it comes to golf. For the past thirty years, I've essentially had to organize my golf life by myself. I've picked up tips wherever I could find them. Pre-internet, I had to wait each month for the new *Golf Digest* and *Golf Magazine* to hit the news-stand. Finally, once the internet and social media emerged, I could watch all the YouTube videos, Instagram posts, and TikTok videos I wanted—going down endless rabbit holes to learn about golf. I have played in countless tournaments around the world, and I've taken hundreds and hundreds of golf lessons (I don't think I want to add them up because I may have broken a thousand). Yet I'm still searching. No one has ever given me that complete story. From the beginning, I sensed there was something more to golf.

No one has ever broken it down for me and said something like: "Mike, there are three parts to golf. There's your golf swing (technique). There's literally how you play golf. And then there are the social aspects of golf, including networking. Here is how they all come together."

The other thing no one ever explained to me was the vocabulary of golf. There are games within games that you play on the golf course. There are virtual golf leagues that exist only in simulator golf. There are so many different places and ways that you can practice golf: 1) On the driving range where you can practice your long game, 2) in short game areas where you can practice your chipping, and 3) on the putting green where you putt. And now in simulators, you can practice any part of your game, anywhere, and the ball always comes back to you, no matter where you hit it.

Networking has been a crucial aspect of golf. I'd always heard that business gets done on the golf course, and that golf networks are the strongest networks, and you really have to break into those. But where are these golf networks? Who's in these golf networks? How do you create these golf networks? Where's the business that's getting done in these deals?

Like many people, I went into golf thinking, *I want to play, I want to be involved in golf.* But I was ignorant about how any of it happened. Nobody laid the complete picture out for me. Golf pros will all teach you something about your golf swing. Who teaches the other parts?

I've been schooled about my swing by the best. But I also wanted golf to create community and enhance my social life (I had moved to

New York City from Chicago when I was still in college; when I later married, my wife, Marcela, was from Buenos Aires, and we needed to meet people). I saw golf as a way to have an amazing relationship with my wife, with my children, and with my friends. It wasn't just about the game of golf. It was about all the things that were around golf, with golf at the center. It was what golf allowed me to do, and the person it helped me become.

In fact, through golf, I serendipitously met Dick Ravitch, one of my most important mentors, friends, and life heroes. We were both taking lessons with golf instructor Debbie Doniger. She thought we were a perfect pair because we both liked politics and had similar golf games. She neglected to mention that Dick was thirty-five years older than me, had run the New York City Metropolitan Transportation Authority, and had also led the Major League Baseball Players Association. I thought I was playing a fun game with a new person. It became so much more than that. Over time, my wife, Marcela, and I became regular partners with Dick and his wife, Kathy, and stayed with them on weekends in the Hamptons. When we golfed, we had a lot to talk about in between holes.

The point of this book is to apply the lessons I've learned as a researcher to golf so that more people can use it to enhance their lives. I won't be teaching you how to swing your club any better, or how to become a better golfer from a score perspective—although the pros I talk to are full of valuable advice. But I will help make you a better golfer from an enjoyment and an enhancement perspective. By the time you finish this book, I hope that you will feel about golf the way I do. I can't imagine a life in which golf is not an integral part.

For those of you who are golf curious, I will give it to you straight in one place. I will try to anticipate all your questions about golf—give you checklists for when you play, teach you about the language of golf and include terms and definitions so you are confident when you start.

My goal is to eradicate golf intimidation. That process starts with cutting through the negative myths surrounding golf. I can't think of any sport where there is so much confusion between professional golf that we see on TV—watching greats like Tiger Woods, Phil Mickelson, Scottie Scheffler, Nelly Korda, Annika Sorenstam, or Michelle Wie West—and the golf we play ourselves. That confusion is deliberate. Professional golf and our golf are played in the same places, on the same courses. We use the same clubs and the same balls. We even wear the same clothes as professional golfers.

Let's clear this up. Amateur golf, club golf, league golfing, couples golf, and family golf are not all the same.

Yes, we can go to the same courses as the greats, and we can even duplicate shots hit by Tiger, Phil, Scottie, Annika, Nelly, or Michelle. The magic of doing what they did makes it all come alive.

In this book I want to capture some of that magic and reveal the common value system of golf. Explore both the norms and the outliers. Many people have said, "You can judge someone's character on the golf course." It might be the way they golf. But it's just the idea that when you're with someone for four hours, you can get to know that person's character. Why does networking happen on the golf course? Because in a four-hour round, you're golfing for ten minutes. What are you doing the other 230 minutes? You're talking. You're chatting. You're getting to know each other in an environment where you can't be on your device the whole time. This is what makes golf special. It's a big part of the reason that golf will change you.

PART 1

THE PROMISE
OF GOLF

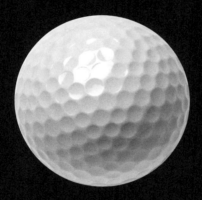

GOLF SAVED MY LIFE

Despite growing up next to the iconic Chicago Park District Golf Course on Chicago's Lake Shore Drive, I'd never swung a golf club before my early twenties.

I started my career working at a company called Penn + Schoen in New York City. P+S was a political polling firm led by Mark Penn and Douglas Schoen that originally attracted public attention working for an audacious congressman named Ed Koch who wanted to be mayor of New York City.

Located on a second-story walk-up above a McDonald's on Third Avenue, the P+S office was a cross between a campaign headquarters and a college newspaper office. It was dark, dusty, and full of bankers boxes stacked with papers thrown everywhere. The office was narrow and went from west to east so there was natural sunlight in the front offices, but there were no other windows going toward the back other than looking out at the fire escape. I would describe it as the office equivalent of a Las Vegas casino. No sense if it was day or night outside. Sunny or raining. We had no idea. And it was perfectly designed that way.

The back half of the office was set up as a phone bank. It had ten folding tables configured in a U shape. Each table had six dialing stations consisting of a push button table phone and an ashtray.

At 5:00 p.m. every afternoon, between forty and fifty people arrived at the phone bank and began the work of dialing randomly generated phone numbers in all parts of the country and interviewing people from questionnaires. Hundreds of households were called each night until around midnight, if we were calling out to the West Coast.

The cacophony of the interviewers talking with their varied accents—Brooklyn, Bronx, Manhattan, New Jersey, Queens, Staten Island, and other accents from around the world—was mind-numbing and beautiful all at once. It was New York City, and I was so happy to be in the middle of it.

And then there was the smoke. Lots and lots of smoke, with very little ventilation. Those were the days when people were allowed to smoke indoors, and they smoked everywhere—at their desks, in the hallway, in the bathrooms, in the stairways. It reminded me of growing up in Chicago when my mother would smoke in the car with the windows rolled up because it was so cold. I'm sure if she had known the risks of secondhand smoke, she would have never done it, but this was the age of blissful ignorance (except in the tobacco industry).

I'd been working at P+S for two years when I began to get sick. I was worn out and developing irritable bowel syndrome. One day my boss Mark looked at me and said, "We need to get you to a doctor." He took me to his brother Deane in Fort Lee, New Jersey, who was a gastroenterologist. He did tests, diagnosed me, and said, "Mike needs a vacation." That was his prescription. (Full disclosure: Dr. Deane was married to my father's sister, Susan Penn, who helped me get my initial internship at P+S, for which I am forever grateful.)

"What?!" Mark was flabbergasted. There was no concept of vacation in those days, especially at a firm like P+S. But Dr. Deane was insistent, so Mark reluctantly agreed. When we got back to the Third Avenue office, Mark told Doug, who said, "Okay, I have a Delta voucher for a free round trip anywhere."

This annoyed Mark. "Who are you?" he barked at Doug. "Are you Santa Claus giving Mike a plane voucher?" But it stuck. I got the voucher. At the time my mother and her husband, Greg, were going to Sanibel Island, a beautiful West Coast Florida waterfront community, so I decided to go with them. Mom and Greg had been going to Sanibel for years and I was curious.

I had a vague idea that I was there to relax, but I really didn't know how. I was pretty keyed up in those days and had grown up in a family that was anti-vacation. My father's motto was, "If you're not in the hospital, you're going to work or school."

But Greg was different from my dad. Greg knew the power of sports to connect people. He owned a chain of neighborhood sporting goods stores in the northwest suburbs of Chicago that specialized in all sports, particularly skiing. But Greg's passion was golf.

One day on Sanibel, Greg took my mom and me to a driving range. I thought I was going to watch him hit balls. Kind of boring. And then he handed me a club. "Try it," he encouraged me. So, I did. I put a tee in the ground, balanced a golf ball on top, and swung this enormous driver called the "Big Whale." And I crushed it. The ball went high and in the air. The adrenaline flew through my body, and the dopamine rushed to my brain. From that first swing, I knew I was a golfer.

This was the sport for me! It meshed perfectly with my personality and inner life in a way nothing ever had before. It allowed me to get into my head, to practice, to be comfortable, to have control, to be part of a world that was new to me. And it got me away from work. In those days there were no cell phones to tether you to work wherever you were. You were tethered to work by being in the office, and for me that meant long hours, often into the night. Golf was an escape from all that. And I began to heal. Freed from the smoke-filled office, out in the fresh air, communing with friends and colleagues as we hit our golf balls across the fairways, I could feel my health returning and my spirits lifting. I hadn't realized just how trapped I'd felt, how burned out and miserable. That's why I can say that golf saved my life.

Golf became a lifelong passion. When Marcela and I got married, we decided that golf was going to be a sport we did together, as well as individually. It became an incredible relationship glue, which we then passed on to both our children, Matthew and Isabella.

I mean it when I say that you really get to know people on the golf course. You see their character, you see how they keep their composure, how they interact with others. It's very social. There's an etiquette to golf, no matter what kind of golf you're playing, that allows you to interact in a more cordial, collegial way. Golf takes down the barriers and enables people to be authentic. There's nothing more authentic than swinging a golf club. You're out there, you can't hide it. You instantly see the result. *Did the ball go up? Did it go in the hole?* And it doesn't matter much after that. Golfers don't care about your score when you play with them. They just want to know how you played. Did you play fast? Were you pleasant to be with? Did you want to engage?

Golf changed my entire perspective on the world. I'm not exaggerating. I'm a happy man, and I owe a lot of that happiness to the gift golf has given me.

THE GOLDEN THREAD

Golf is the golden thread that weaves my professional life and my personal life together. Over the years, I have traveled to more than eighty countries on seven continents, worked for some of the most fascinating brands, including Airbnb, Meta (Facebook), Shell, BP, BlackBerry, OpenAI, the NHL, and Estée Lauder Companies, advised political candidates, including senators, mayors, and presidents, and been part of the Young Presidents Organization for more than twenty-five years. Golf unites my different worlds.

Golf is so much more than just playing a game. For me, golf is the social glue—engaging with clients, with couples, with friends, with family. A common bond is our passion for golfing. As golfers, we find that we spend more time together, we share values, and we share interests.

Even when we have nothing particularly scintillating to say to one another, we can speak golf. *Good shot, great par, tough lie*—are all bonding moments. Golf can break the ice and bring people together. And maybe that is why golf works so well. It contains built-in ice breakers.

> ## The best I can hope for is that people said, "I knew Steve Gilbert. He was fun to play with."
>
> —STEVE GILBERT,
> Founder and Chairman of the Board, Gilbert Equity Partners LP

LIFE'S GREAT MOMENTS

Life's great moments can be celebrated around golf. The most meaningful and emotional golf tournament I've ever played was the 2022 Bo Open, named after my son Matthew's beautiful English bulldog, as part of his wedding weekend over Labor Day.

Matthew and his fiancée, Kristyn, had planned their wedding for a long weekend when they could bring their friends and family together to play golf, hang out, relax, and celebrate. This weekend had it all—a Saturday afternoon pool party for Matthew's twenty-eighth birthday complete with Philadelphia Mummers Parade bands, Saturday night rehearsal dinner, and the all-evening wedding on Sunday.

Matthew and Kristyn decided that starting their three-day wedding weekend with a golf tournament was the perfect way to get everyone on the same page—parents and relatives on both sides, friends on both sides, and the wedding party. Creating groups of golfers, pairings/teams, printing special golf shirts and golf balls, with an open bar at the end got everyone in the right frame of mind. Not to mention a "Bo Cup" to celebrate and drink from to kick off the festivities.

I was paired with Kristyn's mother, Deb, which was amazing because it was two days before her daughter's wedding, and she was so busy, but here she was playing golf! She was relaxed, funny, and hitting the ball well. I learned that Deb is cool as a cucumber under pressure and calm as can be, even with so much going on in her mind. She can compartmentalize so well. I was a wreck, full of nerves. As the father of the groom, I had a lot to learn about grace under pressure from the mother of the bride, and I learned it on the golf course.

After nine holes of golf at the Bo Open, the wedding party had come together. Any separation between those in the wedding party, the families of the kids getting married, and the friends of the bride versus the groom completely disappeared. *We were all just golfers.*

It was brilliant!

A word about Bo, for whom this iconic event was named.

OUR FOUR-LEGGED MASCOT

The pandemic brought about some unexpected bonding experiences both on and off the golf course. While our kids were growing up, Marcela and I had a very strict no-dog rule. We thought with our crazy schedules and my traveling, adding a dog to the mix would be overload.

Of course, as soon as both kids moved out of our house, they both adopted dogs. Isabella chose a fun corgi/Chihuahua rescue dog. Chi-Chi, who lived with Isabella in her apartment in West Hollywood and then in many other apartments in Los Angeles with a brief stop in New York. Isabella likes apartment living, and Chi-Chi goes with the flow and is happy anywhere as long as he's with Isa.

Matthew was working in Greenwich, Connecticut, and during the pandemic, he lived with us. He decided he wanted to adopt an English bulldog. He named him Bo after the inscrutable UK prime minister. Since Matt was living at home, Marcela and I suddenly had a dog.

I was having déjà vu moments having Bo at home as a puppy. It reminded me of when Matthew was born and came home. I had never had a puppy before—just as I'd never had a child before Matthew—so I didn't have a clue what it would be like. No manual or playbook. I just knew that he was incredibly cute and fun to play with. And sometimes, a pain but that will have to be my next book.

Matthew and Bo became inseparable during the pandemic. As Matthew started playing golf every day, he would bring Bo with him on the golf course at Waccabuc Country Club for exercise and as a companion. The two of them became fixtures on the golf course. Bo liked being outside and walking with Matt. Matt enjoyed the company. And the other golfers smiled as they watched a boy (twenty-six!) and his dog on the course walking side by side.

The love culminated with the Bo Open. For me there was the satisfaction of watching Matthew and Kristyn begin their marriage with a shared activity that would enhance their lives, just as Marcela and I had done. The Bo Open symbolized the decades of fun and closeness they could achieve, surrounded by people who love them. It doesn't get any better than that.

IS GOLF RIGHT FOR YOU?

Let's start with a few questions to see if golf is right for you.

Do you like to be with people? Golf is a social sport. You can play with friends, family, and business associates. You can bond, network, build relationships, and even fall in love. Trust is built on the golf course. *Can I do a deal with this person? Is this someone I enjoy being around?*

Do you like the thrill of success? The thrill of success in golf lies in its inherent challenge. Each swing, putt, or strategic decision becomes a personal conquest against golf's unpredictable elements and one's own limitations. There is an exhilarating sense of achievement with golf. And the results are instant. Did the ball go up into the air? Did the putt go into the hole?

Do you enjoy being in great places? Golf is played everywhere. Wonderful golf courses are in the best locations—beautiful natural settings, the great outdoors, where you may even encounter wildlife. Or amazing bars that have golf simulators playing during happy hours. Topgolf has seventy-seven locations in the United States and six countries around the world, offering the atmosphere and sensation of golf in a high-tech space. One of my favorite simulators is my winter course at the Vail Country Club in Avon, Colorado.

Do you like challenges? Golf is as much a mental game as it is physical. It requires concentration, strategy, and patience. Playing regularly can sharpen focus and decision-making skills while reducing stress and increasing relaxation.

Do you want a sport you can play for the rest of your life? Golf is a sport that you can play at almost any age. It is not uncommon to see people playing into their eighties or nineties. This makes it a wonderful sport for longevity and continuous enjoyment.

Do you want to improve your fitness while playing a sport that engages your mind? Playing golf will improve your cardiovascular health as you walk five-plus miles per round across varied terrains, a low-intensity exercise ideal for fat burning. The game's strategic demands also engage the mind, providing mental distraction and making it fun. You don't have to watch Netflix while you're golfing.

Do you want to enjoy off-site ways to get to know, build trust, and have fun with your colleagues? Golf is a great sport to do with work colleagues. It teaches you a lot about each other, even before you begin chatting. It also dissolves layers of authority and puts everyone on the same level playing field.

Are you looking for experiential ways to mentor and lead others? Golf teaches great values. It is a character-building exercise. Self-refereeing requires authenticity, honesty, and emotional control. The game itself is a laboratory for positive life skills such as generosity, humility, humor, kindness, and friendship.

Are you looking for new ways to express yourself? Modern golf is full of opportunities for self-expression, most notably through the expanding field of golf fashion. Gone is the staid, rigid era of country-club uniformity. Golf is a bright new world that encourages you to be yourself.

Do you want new ways to support your community? Golf is ideal for community building and can provide a venue for community support and charitable endeavors. Golf tournaments are often used for charity fundraisers. According to the National Golf Foundation, in 2023 golf was the vehicle for raising $4.6 billion for causes.

Are you interested in adding variety to your life? Golf has an unusual level of flexibility. You can do it by yourself, in groups, and with all types of games. There is not just one way to play golf.

If you answered yes to these questions, golf is the sport for you. I am going to teach you how you can enjoy it to its fullest.

My worst day of golf with friends is still one of the best days of my life.

—JAY HASS,
General Partner, Alley Corp.

LET'S BUST THE MYTHS

As popular as golf is, it's also perceived by many as impossible for them, with multiple barriers to playing. I'm here to tell you that most of these so-called barriers are nonexistent. Let's bust those myths.

• MYTH •
GOLF IS TOO EXPENSIVE

It has never been cheaper to play golf than it is today. With the growth of golf in simulators in restaurants and bars and locations like Topgolf, it can now be played by the hour with clubs and instruction included. And although the expansion of golf has meant some increase in fees on courses, according to the National Golf Foundation, the average fee for eighteen holes at a public course is still only $37. That's comparable to the average workout class such as SoulCycle.

Many people are put off by the costly equipment. But there are plenty of rental opportunities and a strong secondary market for golf equipment that slash the cost.

• MYTH •
IT TAKES TOO LONG TO PLAY GOLF

Golf has evolved to offer many different golf locations from golf simulators at bars, studios, and Topgolf, and golf courses around the world. These alternatives provide many options with a range of time commitments allowing people to choose what fits their schedules. By the way, one of the biggest trends going right now is the nine-hole game versus playing eighteen holes. At around ninety minutes to two hours, nine holes is still a commitment, but a fraction of the four hours you'll spend on the golf course for eighteen holes.

• MYTH •
GOLF IS TOO HARD

With the variety of formats, courses, indoor/outdoor venues, and equipment, it's easy to find the right type of golf for your needs. With equipment enhancements, golf can better adapt to your strengths and weaknesses. It's a whole new ballgame.

• MYTH •
GOLF IS AN ELITE SPORT

Golf has been democratized. And it is my mission to make it even more open and inclusive. Golf is for everyone—that's how it started in Scotland, and that's how it should be now. There are many options for golf: leagues, learning programs, entertainment venues, and so on. A powerful movement is underway to get kids from all socioeconomic backgrounds playing golf earlier in their life, with better access to golf courses and golf instructors.

• MYTH •
GOLF IS FOR RETIREES

While the stereotype of serene greens and a leisurely pace might give an impression that golf is for retired people, the reality of golf is that it appeals to all ages in all locations. Increasingly, golf is for millennials, Gen Z, and even Gen Alpha.

Golf can be played anywhere, anytime, by anyone. The excitement of sounds, noises, and lights at Topgolf or Five Iron Golf can make for a wonderful night out with friends or a date night. The golf course was a pandemic safe haven for many people of all ages. Take a cue from Tiger Woods's family. Fourteen-year-old Charlie Woods is quickly stepping in his father's footsteps. He won a significant junior tournament in September 2023, with Dad serving as caddie.

• MYTH •
THERE'S NO ACCESS TO A GOLF COURSE

Golf is everywhere. Golf can be played and practiced in simulators, driving ranges, and even on video games. There are no limitations to golf other than the commitment it takes to get started. There are more golf courses than Starbucks—17,000 in the United States and 38,000 worldwide.

• MYTH •
GOLF IS STUCK IN THE PAST
AND TAKES ITSELF TOO SERIOUSLY

The modern era of golf is witnessing a cultural shift—music on the golf course, modification and even elimination of dress codes, and high-tech apps on your phone to know distances and keep score. At Michael Jordan's golf course, Grove XXIII (yes, his signature number 23 jersey), the golf carts travel up to thirty-five miles an hour, the caddies ride on golf scooters so they can stay ahead of golfers, drones deliver beer and food to players on the course, and, of course, there is no dress code.

GOLF IS INTIMIDATING

In my interviews with people who want to play golf but haven't, I repeatedly hear about how intimidated they feel. The rules, the dress, the game—they're afraid of being embarrassed. But increasingly there's a different side of golf on display—the side that emphasizes fun and camaraderie. That doesn't mean skills aren't important, just that players can relax in a humiliation-free zone.

GOOD GOLFERS ONLY WANT TO GOLF WITH GOOD GOLFERS

To the contrary, golf is unusually inclusive as sports go. There is always an effort to bring new people into the game. And there tends to be a lot of tolerance, because everyone has experienced being a newbie. If that weren't the case, I wouldn't be writing this book and I wouldn't have encouraged so many people to join the sport.

GOLFERS ARE FULL OF EXCUSES ABOUT WHY THEIR SHOT WENT WRONG

This is actually not a myth, it's true. Golfers are full of excuses—the wind, the lie, the noise, they didn't feel right, everyone and everything is at fault except themselves. That's what makes golf so fun. It is never your fault.

10 WAYS
GOLF WILL CHANGE YOUR LIFE

1. Gives you focus.
2. Enhances your relationships.
3. Makes you more social.
4. Grows your business/network.
5. Supports your causes.
6. Allows you to spend more time outdoors.
7. Helps you lose weight.
8. Enhances your energy.
9. Introduces you to a larger community.
10. Lets you discover and explore new places.

AN OPEN INVITATION

Stephen Curry is a full-fledged celebrity—the point guard for the Golden State Warriors.

As I was writing this in 2024, he was heading to Paris for his first Olympic Games at the age of thirty-six. That outing turned into a spectacular performance that stunned the world and won the American basketball team the gold medal. Curry is definitely a hero on the court, but he holds that title off the court as well.

Curry has always reached out to those who might not have had opportunities to excel. In 2019 he created the lifestyle brand UNDERRATED to create opportunities for young athletes who might not have had a way to get into the sport. It became his passion off the court. For those who think that golf is off-limits to them, and that the barriers are too high, Curry is there to make a case to the contrary. The name of his brand says it all: For those who were underrated and shut out, Curry is issuing an open invitation to join the game.

I spoke with Jason Richards, director of athletic operations for UNDERRATED. He told me that Curry began thinking about a golf outreach during the pandemic. "Everything Stephen does, he wants to make an impact in some manner," Jason said. "It's not about him. It's about how can he change the world for the better, and his North Star was creating a junior golf tour. I think it's been unbelievable to be honest. Even Jordan said it—the platform that Stephen has, and how he's leaning into the game of golf is something that a lot of golfers can't do just because they don't have that following. And when you have Stephen, for whom golf is a true passion, it's electrifying. Some people might say that Stephen likes golf more than basketball."

From the start, Curry's purpose was for sports to better represent what society looks like. "There's a lot of underrepresentation in the game of golf," Jason said. "So, Stephen began to ask, how do we create a space? A platform?"

He noted that Curry wanted to address people specifically in the black and brown communities that are significantly underrepresented in golf. The barriers to entry can be extreme—not just the expense, but also the comfort on the course. So, Curry created a tour to give those underrepresented kids access. His organization takes on the financial burden to give these kids access to private courses and new opportunities. They receive scholarships. But it's about more than just golf. Golf is the entrée into larger life lessons.

"It's about how to build the whole human, for professional life," Jason said. "We have panels where people from the business community come and speak to our kids, not necessarily in golf, but outside of golf, and how golf can translate so much in a professional way. You'll hear

Stephen say this a lot, that golf is just a vehicle to give these kids an opportunity for success in life. And a big part of that is the networking relationships they build."

That network is built from the ground up on the tour. "We didn't know when we built this tour that we were going to create a family. And it's really cool to see because these kids are now friends. Their parents are now friends. They've told us that, before UNDERRATED, they'd go to junior tours, and they might see a couple people of color and get a wave and a hello. But now they're bonding and spending time together."

> ## When you have Stephen [Curry], for whom golf is a true passion, it's electrifying. Some people might say that Stephen likes golf more than basketball.
>
> —JASON RICHARDS,
> describing basketball star
> Stephen Curry's love of golf

Here's another surprising breakthrough. Jason told me: "Most of our elite golfers are young females. We had Ashley Shaw, who's fifteen and played an LPGA event. We had Róisin Scanlon, who's our Curry Cup champion from England—also fifteen. It is extremely impressive how dedicated they are to their craft, and how extremely confident these young women are. There are hundreds of people watching them play, and they're performing at a top level. It's great to see."

Listening to Jason describe this scenario, I reflected on my own experience with golf, and beyond that the purpose of writing this book—to show people how golf could create the strongest relationships of your life and enhance your life in so many ways. And Stephen Curry has created an avenue for that life-changing dynamic to occur for those who were traditionally excluded from the game of golf. There's now an open invitation for them to play.

· 3 ·

THE PANDEMIC PLAY

One of the best examples of the intersection of my professional and golf lives occurred during the pandemic. Golf was a silver lining for many people in those troubled times. It certainly was for me, my family, and many of my friends. But for most of 2020 and going into 2021, it stayed very local.

While we were still working remotely and doing most meetings by Zoom, I was going stir-crazy. I was that guy George Clooney played in the movie *Up in the Air*. I had flown more than ten million miles in my career, and being trapped inside was driving me insane.

I needed to get out.

In the spring of 2021, I traveled to San Francisco to visit my friend and former client, Matt Middlebrook. The sole purpose of the trip was to play golf. And I was ready!

Matt and I first got to know each other in 2012 when he worked in Los Angeles for Caruso Affiliated as vice president of development. We worked on a number of projects at Caruso, but the one fixed appointment we made before and after our meetings was to talk about golf. Matt had caught the golf bug when he lived in Washington, DC, and it stuck with him when he was the Los Angeles deputy mayor under James Hahn.

Over the years, Matt moved on to work at Airbnb in San Francisco. We kept in touch on a personal and a professional basis. Matt introduced me to clients at Airbnb, and we did projects for them as they skillfully managed the pandemic. It was a time when Airbnb's back was against the wall as travel stopped for a time. Then suddenly, when things opened back up, travelers preferred Airbnb over hotels for its safety and sanitization polices. Essentially, Airbnb won the pandemic.

When we worked together at Caruso, Matt was in the process of joining the Olympic Club, an iconic golf club in San Francisco with an epic waitlist—maybe ten-plus years. This course had hosted several US Opens. And it was certainly on my bucket list of courses to play. By the time Matt worked at Airbnb, he was a member. I was ready to join him.

So Matt and I made a wild pandemic plan. I would fly to San Francisco, we would play two rounds of golf in one day, and then I would fly back to New York City. There were two courses that I was obsessed with playing in San Francisco—the Olympic Club and Harding Park, a public course that had just recently hosted the PGA Championship during the pandemic with no crowds. Two iconic golf courses separated by a bay.

What made our plan unusual was that no one was traveling in those days. The airplane flying from New York to San Francisco was empty, and I had to wear a mask the whole way. The hotel I stayed in had contactless everything and looked like a ghost town. No one was having drinks in the lobby, there was no room service or housekeeping, only half of the lights were on, and only one person at a time could ride in the elevator. It was eerie.

But during the pandemic, golf was it. It was the safe sport that was played outside with natural social distancing. A gentle breeze and a little fog in San Francisco made it perfect.

And here it was that Matt and I would spend the next eleven hours together golfing. Catching up, talking about current affairs, learning about each other's kids. In between rounds of golf, we stopped at a delicatessen and ate outside at a table in the parking lot. (As a note, there were also no golf carts, so Matt and I ended up using pushcarts for twelve-plus miles of hilly San Francisco terrain. I definitely slept on the ride back!)

While we played golf, everything seemed back to normal. Two guys playing golf, hanging out, and forgetting about the chaos around us. That's the most important thing about this story. Sure, we played golf. But I can't tell you what I scored or even how I played. I just remember Matt and I hanging out, catching up, and feeling normal.

THE QUARANTINE RELIEVER

Golf gained momentum in the pandemic because it allowed people to have human connections, to be with others outside of their pod, to feel part of a group, and to break out of the crushing isolation.

I've heard a lot from many people, particularly women and millennials, that the pandemic opened their eyes to the benefits of golf and why they should play it. The numbers bear that out. According to the National Golf Foundation, more than 800,000 women and girls started playing golf during the pandemic, the largest cohort to increase its numbers during that period. That represented a 15 percent increase, compared to 2 percent for men. Junior teams found the number of girls increasing from 14 percent of junior golfers to 38 percent.

Why such a rise? The pandemic was a quarantine beater. It had everything you needed during the pandemic:

- An outdoor venue
- Natural social distancing
- No touching

- Being with people safely
- Having fun and breaking out of screen-dependent boredom

In addition, it provided great exercise. Fresh air. The ability to enjoy parts of life every day that had been limited to weekends, days off, and special occasions. Golf became something that people could do every day to break the isolation and monotony. During the pandemic and quarantine, golf allowed people to see, feel, hear, and spend time connecting with others—often on a deeper level than they'd experienced before. Who knew that golf would be the silver lining of a very tough time?

Martin Granda, head golf pro at Waccabuc Country Club, spoke about the impressive influx of new players that arrived during the pandemic. "A large percentage of them were beginners—people who had never played golf," he told me. "People wanted to be outside. Golf suddenly looked fun to them. The majority were women. And more interesting, a lot of members joined who were in their sixties and playing golf for the first time. It's not easy to learn golf at sixty. It's tough!" But that's what happened. And the new influx reenergized golf clubs across the country. Suddenly, because of the pandemic, golf had momentum.

4

THE MOMENTUM OF GOLF

My initial interest in playing golf came from the strong sense that golf was where the action was. I understood that there was power in golf—the mastery of the swing, the social connections that are made and the professional opportunities it builds. I wanted to be a part of it, and I was not alone. I realized that many people felt left out of golf, because they just didn't understand it, felt the barriers to entry were too high, or just didn't know how to get started.

Maybe that was once true, but it isn't true now.

Today, golf is a cultural phenomenon that is sweeping the world. Never has the game been more popular with more types of people playing in more diverse settings. Golf is big business, with $84 billion spent annually. The language of golf is more widely spoken and understood than any other language in the world.

Golf is not new. It has been around for hundreds of years with an origin story dating back to the early fifteenth century in Scotland at the Old Course at St. Andrews—a course you can still play today. Golf has been part of popular culture for decades. There has always been a fascination with golf, its rituals and players. It's featured in popular movies, whether a comedy classic like *Caddyshack*, starring Bill Murray, Rodney

Dangerfield, and Chevy Chase, or Adam Sandler's *Happy Gilmore*, a morality tale like Robert Redford's *The Legend of Bagger Vance*, or a comeback story, like Kevin Costner's in *Tin Cup*.

Even so, I think many people have shied away from golf because, for the past century, it has been a sport for the privileged elite. Wealthy people in private country club settings. Exclusionary clubs—men only, whites only, blue blood WASPs only. Later, in response to exclusion, clubs emerged for Catholics only or Jewish people only. That, too, is changing. Golf has never been as diverse as it is today, inviting more people than ever to the playing field—even if that playing field is not a golf green but a Topgolf venue. This explosion of popularity is introducing the game to new generations of players. And they're loving it.

The newly emerging face of golf is absent many of the negative characteristics that are a turnoff to the next generation—namely the baggage of par and the stress of not embarrassing oneself on the course. It also adds new style trends that shake up the traditions.

THE MOMENTUM FACTOR

In my work as an analyst, I've done a serious study of momentum, and in 2020 I published a book on the subject, *Maximum Momentum: How to Get It, How to Keep It.* A lot of people think of momentum as a trend that comes on like a runaway train. In fact, there's a science to momentum, and that's its secret. The science of momentum harkens back to Sir Isaac Newton's laws of motion. The second law states that an object's movement is dependent on two factors: mass (size) and force (velocity). If we apply this science to today's marketplace, something has momentum when it has *mass* (awareness, reach, impressions, conversations, share of market) and *velocity* (excitement and engagement).

How do we apply this science to the momentum of golf? My research showed that there are five drivers of momentum:

DISRUPTION: Turning something upside down. The idea of outsiders coming in and uprooting the status quo used to be a dangerous idea, but today disruption is the signature of progress in many industries and with many cultural markers. The notion that it's time for a change—and often that change comes from outside the box—is a particularly twenty-first-century notion. Everywhere you look, people are learning not to be afraid of disruption.

INNOVATION: Making something new and improved. We live in an era of constant change. It can be scary at times, but mostly it's exciting. The very idea that we are not bound by the old ways, nor stuck with rigid rules, energizes us every day.

POLARIZATION: Competition and conflict. When there's competition and conflict, people care. And when people care, there is momentum. If there is only one way of doing things, people lose interest, and we know that indifference is the kiss of death for a product, a candidate, or a sport.

STICKINESS: Being memorable. The idea of something being "sticky" was introduced in 2007 by Chip and Dan Heath in their bestselling book *Made to Stick: Why Some Ideas Survive and Others Die*. Sticky ideas take hold. They stay in people's minds and affect their behavior.

SOCIAL IMPACT: Finding larger purpose. The desire to have an impact—to influence an aspect of the social network in a positive way—drives much of the momentum we observe. You don't have to work in an area that is plainly about altruism. No matter where you are, if you're making a social impact, you're gaining momentum.

Let's examine golf through these momentum drivers.

DISRUPTION IN GOLF

Golf went from a sport of older, white males to younger people of all races and genders. During quarantine, on my momentum scale (of

1 to 100), golf's momentum surged to 71 in May 2020 (an exceptionally high score), since it was one of a few socially distanced outdoor activities.

As today's golf evolves, signs of disruption are everywhere, from the course to the simulator to every business and culture style around golf. It's no longer viewed as a sport solely for older white men. Examples of how preconceptions of traditional golf are being challenged include:

- Golfcore (a word coined to describe the shift in golf fashion)
- Nine is fine (par 3 course and playing nine holes instead of eighteen)
- Dualies (those who engage in both on-course and off-course forms of golf)

INNOVATION IN GOLF

Simulator golf driven by technological advances has given players the ability to play golf indoors and on grass. These innovations have also sped up playing times, made the game more social, and created a "come as you are" atmosphere. Increasingly, the message around golf is that it's no longer just a country club sport. There's open access, plenty of variety, and everyone is welcome.

POLARIZATION IN GOLF

"Do you golf?" is a question likely to be asked socially and professionally as a way to introduce yourself in a social or work setting. Being a golfer creates its own set of social and business opportunities. In the past, this tended to be an elitist concept and therefore a negative. Those not in the inner circle would watch their colleagues head off to the golf course, knowing that business was being conducted there, but not being invited.

As access has grown and the circle has expanded, a positive polarization has taken hold, as more people clamor to be part of the game. Now the question, "Do you golf?" is an invitation to join. You don't want to get left on the outside.

STICKINESS IN GOLF

The dopamine effect of golf is legendary. Golf can trigger a significant dopamine release in players, contributing to its addictive and rewarding nature. When golfers hit great shots or achieve positive outcomes, they experience a surge of dopamine, the "feel good" neurotransmitter. Once you feel the rush, you want to repeat the experience.

SOCIAL IMPACT IN GOLF

The values of golf promote integrity, discipline, patience, and respect for others. The game of golf fosters community engagement and charitable giving. Increasingly, it has significant social impact by promoting inclusivity and diversity through programs that introduce golf to underrepresented communities.

In my book *Maximum Momentum*, I chose a catchphrase that people could use to determine whether they were on a momentum track. It was: "Are my best days ahead of me or are they behind me?" Apply that question to golf and you'll find that an enormous shift is taking place. Where once golf was a sport in demographic decline, struggling to attract younger, more diverse players, today it is sizzling with excitement, expanding venues, and bringing in new populations. It's reenergized. No question: Golf's best days are ahead. It has momentum.

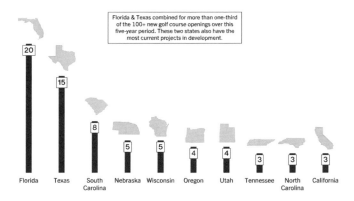

New U.S. Golf Course Openings* by State
(2020-2024)

Florida & Texas combined for more than one-third of the 100+ new golf course openings over this five-year period. These two states also have the most current projects in development.

| 20 | 15 | 8 | 5 | 5 | 4 | 4 | 3 | 3 | 3 |

Florida · Texas · South Carolina · Nebraska · Wisconsin · Oregon · Utah · Tennessee · North Carolina · California

Source: National Golf Foundation Facilities Database
* New course openings include separate 9-holers from a full 18 opening in separate years.
They don't include full reconstructions/rebuilds built on the footprint of a previously existing course
Data herein is member-only and cannot be visually repurposed without permission from NGF.

NGF

A GEN Z POINT OF VIEW

A big question when measuring momentum in golf is whether it can capture the engagement of young people. Many of the experts I've interviewed point to new venues with simulators, experimental formats, and modern styling as attractive to a younger audience, but to find out how young people really feel, I decided to go to the source—my Gen–Z intern Alex Gibani. Alex is a smart young man and, best of all, he has his finger on the pulse of his peers, the Zoomers. And he has the statistics to back up his impressions. When I asked Alex to share his thoughts about golf, he accepted the challenge enthusiastically, and here's what he had to say. Take it away, Alex:

POV ALEX GIBANI

If you've kept up with the news, you'd be forgiven for thinking that Gen Z and the game of golf are an unlikely partnership. Born between the mid-to-late '90s through the early 2010s, Zoomers are known for their perceived lack of attention spans, addiction to screens, political activism, you know the rest. Not exactly traits commonly associated with a love for the historically conservative game of golf. As someone born in 2001, coming of age at the dawn of the social media era, and graduating high school in the middle of the pandemic, I'm supposed to love football and basketball, video games and Instagram. I'm not supposed to have refined social skills or the attention span to handle a four-hour round of golf. And to be completely honest, I don't.

Growing up, I'd always wanted to try golf, but stuffy golf courses, $100-plus rounds, and a general fear of absolutely embarrassing myself kept me far away. I didn't golf; I played hockey. But many of my friends golfed, and as I've gotten older and my hockey career has wound down, I have found myself longing to join my friends on the course. To have that common ground in a conversation when somebody looks at me and asks me what my handicap is and not politely tell them that, well, I suck. This basically makes me the definition for *latent demand* in golf, which is somebody who doesn't play golf but who's very interested in playing now. And I am increasingly not alone. Since the beginning of the pandemic, latent demand is up nearly seven million people, with the highest percentage age bracket being the six-to-seventeen cohort. Or, in other words, smack dab in the middle of Gen Z.

How could this be? Nearly every trait associated with golf precludes it from being a viable pastime for Gen Z. Short attention spans? An eighteen-hole round typically takes well over four hours. Aversion to going outside? It's impossible to play eighteen rounds indoors. More liberal minded and prone to activism? Try that at a typical golf course. Yet off-course golf participation (simulators) in the six-to-seventeen age bracket has grown 40 percent since 2019, compared to just 2 percent for middle-aged people. Any number of arguments could explain this number, but as a member of Gen Z, my experience is that golf has gained popularity because of off-course venues.

On-course growth since 2019 sits at about 14 percent, while off-course, which includes simulators and hybrid venues such as Topgolf, has grown over 41 percent. The average age of an off-course-only golfer is thirty-two, compared to forty-six years for exclusively on-course golf. It's clear from this that off-course golf sits at the intersection of an entirely new industry but is also the future of the game. Over 65 percent of on-course beginners are coming to the game with some sort of off-course experience. At least 10 percent of green-grass golfers credit the beginning of their golf journey to places like Topgolf. It's acting as both a different way to play the game as well as a feeder to on-course golf. For me, personally, this is how I plan on getting into the game. Rather than ponying up precious cash to embarrass myself on a course, I could go with my friends and have a good time at Topgolf while also working on my game. The numbers back this up as well, with 95 percent of people saying that it provides a more approachable way to try golf and over 75 percent stating that it helped them realize that they could be comfortable at a golf course.

Golf's reputation as a stuffy game for old people is rapidly changing. While I've known this my whole life, it's only because

I grew up in an area where golf is a common pastime. That this is becoming a trend among members of my generation from different areas is telling of a broader national shift. In 2013 only 17 percent of eighteen-to-thirty-four-year-olds described golf favorably, where just ten years later that number is 30 percent. It's not universal approval, but it's a trend that is echoed across every age group. Personally, I think that social media is a huge reason for this. The stereotype that my generation gets nearly all of its opinions through social media has a myriad of negative effects, but it seems that golf has bucked that trend. For example, recently my friends have become obsessed with a streamer named Sketch, whose signature videos include him wandering around a golf course whacking balls and screaming obscenities into the camera. His Instagram account has over a million followers, and one YouTube video of him golfing has over two million views. His catchphrase, "What's up, brother" with a finger pointed to the sky has been adopted by nearly my entire circle. He recently announced the Houston Texans' draft pick on national television. He's entered the cultural mainstream and is dragging golf along with him.

Surveys show that adults engaged with social media have categorically higher perceptions of golf compared with their peers who aren't. More eyeballs, particularly from my generation, are on the game and, based off all available evidence, this can only be a good thing for its growth. I know in my case, seeing someone on Instagram in a T-shirt crushing beers and laughing with his friends looks like a good time.

I'm still a little scared of going out onto the course with my friends. The only green-grass experience I've had was surprising my buddy with a round on the public course in my town, where I used my dad's 1989 3-wood to smash balls into the opposite fairway. If

I were playing with good players on a course like Wee Burn, I'd be embarrassed beyond belief, but I distinctly remember having the best time because, first, I was with my best friends, and second, there was no pressure to succeed. We all stank—and no one cared.

I miss playing with my friends. I miss walking around the green grass and having the best time. And seeing places like Topgolf, where you can go outside, have a few drinks, and smash a couple of balls, gives me hope that I can experience this again. I'm just glad that I'm not alone.

Golf Participation in the U.S.
Key Statistics

vs. '22 | vs. '19 | # New high mark

		vs. '22	vs. '19	
Total Participation	45.0M#	▲9%	▲32%	The total number of golf participants (on- and off-course included), has increased 53% in less than 10 years, up from about 30M total in 2014
Total Off-Course	32.9M#	▲18%	▲41%	Off-course participation has eclipsed on-course in each of the past two years, and more than doubled since 2014 (14.3M)
Total On-Course	26.6M	▲4%	▲14%	2023 marked the sixth straight year that on-course participation has increased, with a net Y.O.Y. gain of 1M being the largest single-year jump since 2001
Beginners	3.4M#	▲3%	▲3%	The number of first-time on-course players reached another high – the fourth straight year of at least 3M newcomers (after averaging 2.6M from 2016 to 2019)
Youth (ages 6-17)	3.5M	▲4%	▲40%	There were more on-course youth golfers in 2023 than any year since 2006; this segment has experienced the largest gains of any age group since 2019 (+40%)
Young Adult (ages 18-34)	6.3M	▲2%	▲4%	The number of young adults playing "green grass" golf has increased for the third consecutive year, and is at its highest point since 2015
Middle-Aged (ages 35-64)	11.4M	▲1%	▲2%	From an age perspective, golf's on-course growth has come primary at the "bookends," although the "middle-aged" cohort has incremented as well
Senior (ages 65+)	5.4M	▲15%	▲17%	The oldest age cohort saw its first meaningful on-course participation increase in the post-Covid era – a net gain of almost 700K golfers
Female	7.0M	▲9%	▲25%	Four straight years of gains have yielded a 1.4M participation increase since 2019 ; females comprise 26% of all on-course golfers – another record high
People of Color	6.1M	▲8%	▲27%	People of color (+1.4M since 2019) now represent 23% of all "green grass" golfers – a new high mark in racial and ethnic representativeness
Latent Demand	22.4M#	▲8%	▲45%	The number of Americans who didn't play on-course golf in the past year but are "very interested" increased by almost 1.5M and reached another new high mark
Rounds Played	531M	▲4%	▲20%	2023 surpassed 2021 (529M) for the most rounds in a single year in U.S. history. It was the fourth straight year with 500M+ rounds played in the U.S.
Avg Rounds Per Golfer	20.0	◄►	▲10%	The increases in rounds played continue to be driven primarily by the most avid and committed golfers playing more frequently than in past years.

THE NEW BRANDING ARENA

We live in an age when your product, service, or other offering is only as good as your branding. When I started investigating the golf world, I found that it was alive with innovation and branding for new audiences. It was a clear sign that the sport was being enlivened and had a healthy future.

RONAN GALVIN
Making Golf Bags as Easy as Sunday Morning

Ronan Galvin, creator of the company Sunday Golf, is an example of the youth and flexibility trend. Ronan's background is in product development and manufacturing. He has invented a unique golf bag, which is so much more than a bag. It's a golf ideology.

First, it's important to note that Ronan was not even a golfer. In fact, he was always turned off by golf. "I played basketball and football growing up," he told me. "Frankly, I shied away from golf. It was too long and too boring." Professionally, he followed a track in product development that led him into the golf industry, but for a long time he wasn't a player.

He avoided playing for as long as he could. Around the office, golf was what people did. The golf course was where they took clients. They'd often ask, "You want to go play?" and he'd always fake being sick or busy. When he was being honest, he'd say: "Dude, I don't even know how to swing a club. There's no way I'm going out with a client and look like an idiot. It would be bad for me professionally."

Then, a few years back, "I got dragged to a par 3 course with my buddies." It wasn't at all what he expected. The Loma Club in San Diego wasn't the buttoned-up, hushed environment he'd been expecting. It was a par 3 course. He saw golfers wearing tank tops and flip-flops. Flip-flops! And there was music playing and everyone looked chill. The longest hole was 130 yards, making it hard to mess up. So, he played, and to his shock he thought, *This is fun!* He was pleasantly surprised. "It was definitely more relatable, more digestible."

He did notice one thing, though. Golfers were lugging their full-sized bags, even when they were only using half their clubs on the par 3 course. His mind cut to the product development possibility, and soon he'd created a prototype for a bag that only held three or four clubs. When he brought his prototype to the course, everyone wanted one. It was a no-brainer.

The name, Sunday Golf, was inspired by the relaxed, easygoing mood that the lighter bag implied. I thought it was genius. I've always thought of Saturday golf as serious business. There you've got your regular games. But Sunday golf is more relaxed; it's like family golf. You've got your kids, your couples, your casual players. That's the Sunday zeitgeist on the course, and Ronan tapped into that. In the process, he has helped create exactly the environment that makes golf work for him. Before, all it had been missing was the fun.

Sunday Golf bags make the sport more accessible. You can imagine men, women, boys, and girls easily walking the course with their tailored bags, happily socializing with their friends and being on the go. It's a nice, inclusive picture.

EARL COOPER
Breaking Barriers and Leading the Way

Eastside Golf, which started in Detroit with roots in East Atlanta, produces a line of unique golf apparel for comfort and style—with a message. Its motto is "Be Authentic." While it celebrates the great black golfers who first broke the color barrier, the emphasis today is not on trying to fit in, but on creating its own cultural dynamics around golf. I was first introduced to Eastside through StockX, which promoted a new trend called GolfCore—creators of new, viral fashion around sports brands in cities like Detroit.

Golf apparel may seem like a sideline, but it has become an essential statement embodying the adoption of the sport by a broader base of young men and women. These players reject the old-fashioned golf uniforms for styles that suit their taste and comfort.

The goal of black creators Olajuwon Ajanaku and Earl Cooper is to collaborate with leading brands such as Nike and Jordan to open the door to a new generation of minority golfers. Their efforts to create awareness and opportunity for black golfers landed them on *Black Enterprise* magazine's "40 Under 40" list.

I spoke with Earl Cooper about Eastside's positioning. We discussed the exclusionary history of the game. "Everybody looks at golf now [in 2024] and asks, 'Where are all the minorities?'" he said. "Well, look, we were just allowed into the place for the first time sixty years ago. The PGA was founded in 1913, so that was fifty-plus years of total exclusion. And the Jim Crow era lingered some after 1962. It wasn't like everyone was opening their arms and saying, 'Come on in.' Maybe legally they couldn't keep us out, but there were a lot of other ways. So, we're still trying to play catch-up."

Earl grew up in Wilmington, Delaware. One day his father saw a flyer for the Urban Youth Golf Program, and he signed Earl up. "There wasn't an instant love affair," Earl told me. He was pretty good at the game, but he didn't feel entirely comfortable. To put it bluntly, "I didn't like it because none of my friends were there."

He stuck with it, though, and by thirteen he was winning locals and competing in regionals. When he started winning big prizes, like a free trip to Walt Disney World, he felt that all the hard practice was worth it. "I finally just said: 'All right. I'm a golfer. I'm talented at this.' It gave me the confidence to say, 'This is what I do.' And I'm very grateful to my parents, specifically my father, who kept me involved."

As he got older, Earl became more aware of the exclusionary side to golf. "We worship exclusivity, the elite nature of the game—the 1 percent everyone aspires to. People talk about the Seminoles . . . Cypress Point." So, how does a game grow when it is steeped in exclusion? The answer is that it doesn't. And Earl's goal is to grow the game. It's the underlying mission of Eastside Golf.

"We want to use our platform in any way we can, on the biggest stages in golf—such as a collaboration with the Jordan brand, sponsoring an invitational in San Diego where the PGA color barrier was first broken by Charles Sifford," he told me.

Earl hopes that Eastside Golf can open the door to educate and create a sense of belonging. Most people know little to nothing about the history of black golf. Who were the leaders? Who broke the barriers? He noted that Tiger Woods named his son after Charles Sifford. "We want to pay homage and use our platform with major brands to look back and talk about the historical significance of blacks and the game."

Eastside Golf is helping to make it happen on the ground in an ever-widening frontier. They sponsored the Eastside Golf Invitational in San Diego, where Sifford played and broke the barrier. "We're very intentional about the way we show up," Earl emphasized. A second event is planned in New Jersey at Liberty National Golf Course. It's scheduled to take place during Fashion Week, which draws culture-oriented crowds to the city. "It'll be a great vibe. We want to give our audience an opportunity to access the types of facilities they might not have experienced. We're bringing cultural inclusion. We want to be ourselves."

That idea resonated with me—being themselves. Not fitting into a golf niche but creating their own arena. And within this arena, the message is one of helping youth apply the values of golf—to better themselves and change their lives.

IGOR REYES
A Clubhouse Michael Jordan–Style

Speaking of creating a different mood on the course, Michael Jordan has figured that out. I spoke to Igor Reyes, president of Nichols Architects (formerly Nichols Brosch Wurst Wolfe & Associates), the architecture firm that designed the clubhouse at Jordan's private golf club, the Grove XXIII.

When the firm was first approached about the project, Igor hesitated. "I'd been an architect for thirty years, working on all kinds of hotel and hospitality projects. This was different. I kept saying to our PR person, 'Do they know that I do not golf?'" Nor did he want to golf. It wasn't his thing. But he'd done a Ritz-Carlton hotel in Jupiter, and Jordan had used the clubhouse there and loved it. Jordan liked the flow and other details of the way it worked. He wanted to talk to the guys who did that clubhouse.

When Igor and his colleagues met with Jordan, they quickly learned that, as Igor put it, "He likes to play golf the way he likes to play golf." That meant a real club atmosphere—music, cigars, breaking some rules here and there, and doing what he likes to do. He's Michael Jordan, so he can do it. He can build his own clubhouse any way he wants it."

His vision was a long way from the old clubhouses with their mahogany wood paneling, marble showers, and muted conversations. "That old school atmosphere was to be avoided for Jordan and his buddies," Igor told me. "Jordan wanted something different, and we just went along with him."

The premise Igor's firm developed was simple: "We basically said: 'Our building has to have the attitude Michael Jordan brought to the basketball court. We'll bring it to the golf course.'"

For one thing, the clubhouse and the course are integrated—the clubhouse is right off the ninth hole. And it's not the old-fashioned mahogany wood style. "Jordan wanted to sit and keep looking at the golf course and not leave the course, avoiding that disconnect," Igor explained. "The clubhouse is basically a covered area with a bar and a large humidor so you can smoke cigars. It has the feeling of a lounge, more than a club. It's a lot less formal, a lot more comfortable, a lot more laid back—so Jordan can feel like he's in his living room with his buddies—completely without hierarchies. It's a hangout spot to play and enjoy the setting, and I have to wonder if this is the future of golf."

What I took away from Igor is that Grove XXIII was redefining the relationship between the clubhouse and the golf course. The clubhouse was no longer designed to keep people out, but to invite people in and let everyone participate. That's what happens when you sit courtside at a basketball game at the United Center. You don't have to be playing in the game to feel part of the action.

STEPHEN AND ERICA MALBON
Who Says You Have to Conform?

Golf's reputation for being old and stuffy is being challenged on every front. What's interesting to me is that the challengers aren't taking on the traditions of golf. They are very much committed to the game. Their point is that it doesn't always have to be done the same way.

A very big trend in marketing is collaborations. Mashing up two brands to see what comes out, such as a Post Malone X Croc. One only needs to check out *Vogue* for a picture of an up-and-coming golf apparel business that is all about the young, hip crowd. Stephen and Erica Malbon count among their fans and customers Justin Bieber and Travis Scott, among others. These are culture leaders who are embracing golf *their* way.

The couple came to the idea of their apparel brand Malbon Golf after many years building companies. Stephen created Frank151, a creative agency and street magazine. Erica is the cofounder of The Now, a hip boutique spa and massage parlor in Los Angeles. As they turned their joint attention to this new challenge, they defined their mission as showing kids they can golf and be cool—and have fun.

"For us, the question is always, what excites us? What are we passionate about?" Erica said. "We saw the opportunity—a golf brand that looks at the sport from a different perspective."

Apparel, they noted, is often the entrée to a deeper engagement in various arenas. And the reach of the internet, especially social media, allows their message to have a wide reach. "Everyone is a fan of someone," Erica pointed out. "And when those people are inspiring young people to play golf and are saying, 'Golf is cool. I love it'—people like Justin Bieber—the young people who look up to them are going to say, 'I do too.'"

Stephen admitted that in his early golf days, working in advertising in New York, he was embarrassed to be a golfer. "The reputation of golf was so stuffy and snooty. So, when we started our company, we did it unapologetically, being true to ourselves. It's okay if you like music, fashion, and art, and you also want to play at Augusta National or Cypress Point or Pine Valley. Where is it written that you have to conform?"

Erica agreed. "At the majority of country clubs, you have to have a collared shirt, you have to tuck it in, you have to wear a belt. If you're a woman, you can't wear a skirt. You have to wear pants. It rubs people the wrong way. I don't want to be told what to wear."

Malbon Golf is leading the way in individuality within the larger arena of golf. "This is how we frame ourselves," Erica said. "We love the game of golf. We love the heritage, the history. We respect the special background. At the same time, we want to infuse a freshness and a stylish perspective. We've worked hard and, as a result, our business is growing, and the sport is growing. The perception of golf is changing. This is what we aspire to—to look back and be able to say, wow, we really did make a big impact on the sport as a whole."

It wasn't easy being nonconformists in a conforming golf world, and the Malbons almost crashed in the beginning. But they were tenacious and kept going because they knew they had a breakthrough. Today, top brands want to do collaborations with them, and they've captured the momentum.

DAVID GAGNON
Making Everyone Feel at Home on the Golf Course

David Gagnon, the director of golf at GlenArbor Golf Club in Bedford Hills, New York, chatted with me about the ways golf is approached these days and what people want from it. He's been with GlenArbor for twenty-two seasons. Like many pros I spoke with, he didn't start out as a golfer. In high school he was attracted to a riskier sport—racing motocross. His mom eventually made him stop because it was too dangerous. So, he started hanging out with his buddy next door, and his buddy's brother played golf. He joined him on the course one day and "went from zero to a hundred" pretty quickly.

He never looked back. It wasn't a conscious decision, but once he started playing, he was hooked. "I love playing the game and I love teaching the game," he told me. "That's never changed for me. I never drive by a golf course that I don't want to play—ever."

David gives a lot of thought to the question, what do golfers really want? "Some people just want to get better as a point of pride. Others want to get better to compete at a higher level. Still others want to get better, so they won't be embarrassed when they play."

> ## I really couldn't care less how good somebody is when I'm playing with them. And most good players feel the same way.
>
> —DAVID GAGNON,
> Director of Golf at GlenArbor, Bedford Hills, New York

And yet, despite this last factor, David will tell you that the biggest misconception of golf is that people care about your score. He laughed at the thought. "I really couldn't care less how good somebody is when I'm playing with them," he said. "And most good players feel the same way." The most important thing is that you are fun to play with and play *fast*.

Imagine how this simple notion could change the way people think about golf—and lower their stress levels.

David has a special place in my personal golf history. He has spent each of the last twenty-two years of his teaching career teaching me. He started with me when I literally could not swing a club. Painstakingly, he has worked with me through all aspects of my game. David lived in Connecticut year round, and during the winter months before they had simulators, I'd have lessons in the outdoor teaching bay at GlenArbor, with the wind blowing in cold. David would be decked out in his winter coat, gloves, and hat as he helped me practice. I was relentless and he never gave up on me. Malcolm Gladwell has said that it takes ten thousand hours to master something. It feels as if I had David there for all ten thousand hours.

I want to emphasize that during those grueling lessons, David was always patient and kind. He had an affirmation strategy. If I hit one out of ten balls correctly, he would say, "That's what I'm talking about." Meanwhile, I knew just how bad the other shots were. David would just say, "Let's get to work." He never asked my score. He always just saw my smile and encouraged me to play more. He knew that if I scheduled a lesson a day after a tournament, it hadn't gone well for me. And in fifteen minutes, he would have the problem fixed.

5

THE CALL OF THE COURSE

When I started to really get into golf, I wanted to find out which were the best golf courses. I didn't know any of the names, so I didn't have the usual golfer's bucket list of places I wanted to play.

At the time there were two golf magazines—*Golf Digest* and *Golf Magazine*. Remember, this was pre-internet. I was an avid reader of both magazines, although half the time I didn't know what they were talking about. I was definitely on a learning curve. They would have sections with tips if you were a 10 handicapper, a 15 handicapper, or a 20 handicapper. I'd read all three and be lost. But each month when I was flying my thirty thousand miles, I was sitting with all the other people in business class reading their golf magazines. Maybe they knew what they were about.

The magazines were structured with cover stories featuring professional golfers who would share insights into their life and the game. They would also feature major tournaments, such as the Masters, the US Open, the British Open, and the PGA tournaments.

I did know something about the US Open Tennis Tournament, because when I was growing up, John McEnroe and Bjorn Borg had epic matches around Labor Day, which I watched on TV. I also remember

Wimbledon because we'd get up early on a Sunday morning to watch. But I didn't remember any equivalent golf games, although I knew the names Arnold Palmer and Jack Nicklaus.

Once I started playing and following golf in the 1990s, I began paying more attention to the various courses. I noticed that most of the tournaments were played at different courses every time—one time in Wisconsin, one time in California, one time in Pennsylvania, one time in Oklahoma, and so on. But the Masters Tournament was always played at the Augusta National Golf Club in Augusta, Georgia.

As I traveled for work, I began to make a point of playing at golf courses in various places. At one point I bought a pegboard from *Golf Magazine* to keep track. The board was a way to keep track, and it was also aspirational. It listed the one hundred top golf courses, and every time you played one, you put a peg in. I set a goal to play as many of the courses as possible. I became a frequent organizer of golf trips with a group of friends, although there were some obvious choices that I skipped. For example, I didn't want to play in Scotland or Ireland because, to be frank, I didn't like to play in the rain. I'm a fair-weather golfer! I like to play in nice conditions.

On our golf trips, we went to the West Coast. We played Bandon Dunes Golf Resort in Oregon; Pebble Beach in Carmel, California; and nearby courses Spyglass Hill and Spanish Bay. I was also working on my pegboard with my YPO group, with the Pinehurst Resort in North Carolina, and the Greenbrier in West Virginia.

THE ULTIMATE PRIZE: AUGUSTA NATIONAL GOLF CLUB

Augusta National Golf Club is like none other—it was number two on my pegboard, but it was the most talked about, most coveted, and most iconic course, and I'd aspired to play there for almost twenty years. I finally had the opportunity in 2004, thanks to my friend and fellow YPO forum mate, Jim. I never could have imagined how much joy and fulfillment would come from playing any golf course, and the experience at Augusta was life changing. Jim's generosity as a member opened this opportunity for me—he'd grown up there; his grandfather and father were members. Now he offered me and two of my best friends (and YPO forum mates), Tony and William, a chance to play in a foursome with him, and I jumped at the chance. Tony and William had played at Augusta before, but this felt more personal. Jim was our friend, our age, in our forum.

As I've mentioned, I wasn't in the habit of watching the Masters Tournament. I can remember my mom's husband, Greg, blocking Masters weekends out and being glued to his sofa on Saturday and Sunday watching the tournament unfold in Augusta. I didn't know much about the history and traditions of Augusta. So, I was a sponge, breathing it all in.

When we arrived at Augusta, we drove down the famous Magnolia Drive with its stunning flowers, and I knew I was somewhere special. I discovered that Augusta reinforces all the elements that make golf unique and beautiful. On this course, one is reminded of the storied traditions of golf, as well as its cultural significance. It is all about the golf experience without distractions. The rules are all about enhancing the experience. Cell phones, golf carts, all distractions, are banned. You're required to play with a caddie, who serves as your ambassador to the incredible club.

But more important, you can feel the presence of the iconic figures who made a mark on this course. President Eisenhower (Ike) in the 1950s who had a cabin on the course dubbed the "Little White House." The great golfer and founder of the Masters, Bobby Jones. Jack Nicklaus, one of the top golfers of all time, who made the sport popular in the sixties and seventies.

You become a part of the course when you play at Augusta. You're one with the experience, with the people in your foursome, with the trees and flowers and blades of grass and the spirit in every cabin. And you also feel connected to the other people playing that day, and to the staff who work there. Everything else in the world outside the course fades into the background.

I was in my comfort zone because I was playing with my closest friends—my go-to buddies I had been golfing with for years. I wasn't intimidated by the course, but I remember hitting my shot on the first tee, and it literally went 45 degrees: I hit my tee shot into the pro shop, which is an impossible shot, but I did it. (This is one of those stories I have been telling myself for so many years that I don't even know if it is true anymore. But I know my first shot was really bad and went someplace to the right where no one had ever seen a ball go. So, I told myself it went in the pro shop. It is not out of the realm of possibility.)

As we played, I learned about "Amen Corner," the section of the course at the eleventh, twelfth, and thirteenth holes, which is known as the most difficult part of the course where a player has to say his prayers. Through these stories, the course came alive for me, and so did our bond of twenty years. We'd taken a photo twenty years earlier, and we re-created it at Augusta, full of the happiness of two decades playing together.

After I played there, my obsession with Augusta didn't abate—it had just started. I'd watch the Masters on TV and realize that this wasn't just another course on my pegboard. It was my happy place where I'd go with my friends to escape the cares of the world. I have returned on numerous occasions for our friendly foursome. Believe me, it's hard to schedule these trips because everyone is so busy. But it's Augusta and we manage.

I love being on the course, in the setting where greats like Phil Mickelson hit their famous shots. I remember one time we reprised a shot Tiger hit on the fifteenth hole, hitting the exact place on the fairway, within five yards of each other, all in a straight line. What a thrill.

There's tradition all around us at Augusta. I've been fortunate to be able to pass the experience to my son, this time as a spectator. He brought his wife to watch the Masters Tournament, and now he's talking about bringing my grandson, Leo. I know it's just a golf course, but it's come to embody so much more for our family.

The anticipation is a constant. I don't know any other place in my life that, as soon as I leave, I want to come back. And for once I don't care about the weather. I just want to be there. I've played Augusta when it's 40 degrees and pouring rain. I've played when it seems like 100 degrees, and I've consumed a full bottle of water on each hole. I've played Augusta when I could not hit a ball that wasn't perfectly straight. I've played when I couldn't hit a ball anywhere close. It didn't matter. The experience was still magical every time.

What Augusta has done better than any place in the world is make community, values, and etiquette count. No matter the game, it's elevated when it takes place at Augusta. When I watched the Augusta National Women's Amateur the week before the Masters, I was so proud of the amateur women—the great play-through challenge and the pressure of playing the course in Masters conditions. I watched the Augusta National Women's Amateur end to end, and I found the amateurs just as interesting as the pros. It's the specialness of the place that makes the difference.

I'm a gearhead, so I bring the latest and greatest technology and drivers every year. For example, one year Nike had square drivers that made a clank that sounded like an aluminum bat when they hit. One year I brought TaylorMade Qi10 drivers.

I also love swag, and I collect hats and shirts. I always buy presents for everyone at Augusta. I've brought Marcela many beautiful quarter zips and T-shirts, but I've never bought anything for myself because, as I see it, Augusta is in my heart. I don't have to wear it.

I understand why so many people want to play on this famous course, but for me it's special because it's where I really learned to appreciate golf with my friends. We have the stories from those trips, and I cherish them and love to pull them out when we're reminiscing.

AUGUSTA MEMORIES

The Masters Tournament has a history of famous golf shots made by legendary golfers that define its history. As we casually play the Augusta National course, the caddies always show us the exact spots where these epic shots were made: Phil Mickelson through the pine straw on thirteen, Tiger Woods chipping in on sixteen, or Bubba Watson hitting his wedge from the trees onto the 10th hole to win the playoff.

Over the years, my friends and I have developed our own memories of legendary shots: William reaching the par 5 fifteenth green in two shots, Tony splashing the perfect bunker shot on the par 3 twelfth hole on Amen Corner, Jim bombing his drive down the seventh fairway, or my birdie on the downhill par 3 fourth hole. These moments are recalled every time we play.

Our bond and our connection with Augusta endures. And every time I leave, I say to myself, "If I never come back, this has been the most amazing golf experience I've ever had." And every time I return, I say, "I can't believe I'm here."

TOMORROW'S GOLF COURSE

I spoke with Don Placek, a golf course designer/architect with Renaissance Golf Design. He's been around golf his entire life. His dad was a golf pro at Lakewood Country Club, a Donald Ross course in Denver, Colorado. When Don was four years old, the family moved from Denver, to a small town in southwest Nebraska where the clubs were more casual. They didn't have rigid rules and dress codes. "What they worried about was how you treated each other, and how much fun you had playing the course," Don said. "That's the atmosphere I grew up in. And the men and women in that little course in McCook, Nebraska, always included me. They didn't just tolerate me, they encouraged me."

> As humans, we gravitate toward stability and predictability. It makes us feel comfortable. But we've discovered for a lot of reasons that golf is way more fun when it isn't the same thing over and over.
>
> —DON PLACEK,
> Golf Course Designer, Renaissance Golf Design

Don cut his teeth on public golf courses. In college he worked for the Colorado Golf Association (CGA), the authority on amateur golf in the state. "Their mission statement was, 'Golf is for everybody.' As a nonprofit, they weren't out to make money. They were committed to making the game accessible, affordable, and sustainable, through junior golf, state amateur events, and developing caddie programs for kids."

As a professional at Renaissance Golf, Don had the opportunity to help design and build what is today CommonGround GC in Denver, reimagining a decommissioned US Air Force base course with renowned golf architect Tom Doak for the CGA.

The grand strategic idea for CommonGround, now home to the CGA and its myriad of public golf programs and so many other courses Don designs is variety and excitement. "As humans, we gravitate toward stability and predictability," Don said. "It makes us feel comfortable. But we've discovered for a lot of reasons that golf is way more fun when it isn't the same thing over and over. Golf can and should be exciting, changeable, and fun. That's what we're tapping into, and in the process, continuing to make golf more available and affordable too. That's the only way to make golf sustainable. Capturing your audience when they're sixty isn't nearly as beneficial as getting them when they are six. We need to captivate them when they are six."

As terrible as the pandemic was, Don saw it as a catalyst for golf. People had to be outside, and they gravitated toward outdoor activities, even if they had never played golf before.

So, how do you get someone hooked on golf? Don considers it a core experience, and he draws recognizable comparisons. "I remember my dad and grandfather taking me fishing for the first time. Baiting my hook, setting the bobber, and casting my line into the pond. Then waiting for the bobber to duck beneath the surface and feeling the 'tug' by the fish! There's nothing like that first 'fish on' experience! Or learning to balance and ride your bike minus the training wheels for the first time. Golf can be like that too—the first time you hit a ball on the face of the club, on the sweet spot, and the ball just *rockets* into the sky, its special and addicting. I want more young people to experience that feeling. And it doesn't have to happen on a driving range. These days it can be at Topgolf, a par 3 course or other venues. Where a swing and a miss is fine. Just laugh and try again—that is until you catch one squarely. After that you could be hooked for life!"

· PART 2 ·

THE SOCIAL
POWER OF GOLF

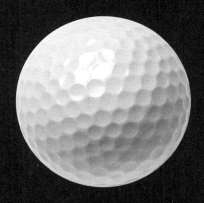

6

GOLF IS MY NETWORK

When Marcela and I got married, we made a commitment to each other that we were going to take up three sports that we could do together. The first sport was tennis. We had both played a little bit of tennis, and we thought it would be a good couples sport and would allow us to meet other couples. We enjoyed going to the US Open together and have done so every year of our marriage. In the first few years, we were consigned to the nosebleed section in nearly the last row. We had a better view of the airplanes landing at LaGuardia than Andre Agassi defeating Pete Sampras.

Our second couple sport was skiing, which we've enjoyed on winter vacations in Colorado. (Before that time, I had only skied once in my life. There aren't that many ski resorts in Chicago. Marcela had more experience in Argentina and Chile.)

Our third sport was golf. At the time, I had just started golfing down in Sanibel with Greg, and Marcela was new to the sport too. But somehow I knew that this could be the equalizer. Golf had long-term potential, and we could do it together. We slowly incorporated golf into our lives. At this point, we were still living in Manhattan, so it was mostly me going to driving ranges when I could or bringing Marcela on vacation in Longboat Key, Florida. Or playing with Greg on visits to Chicago. It was very low-key. Then, in 1998, about seven years into our marriage, we moved from New York City to Westchester County, a northern suburb with a lot of golf courses. Our home was in the hamlet of Waccabuc, situated in the town of Lewisboro, with its own country club and golf course located around the corner from our house. At the time we didn't even think about joining. For one thing, there was a three- to five-year waiting list, and we had to get called up. Second, we didn't really understand how it all worked. And third, the golf course looked huge. I was used to hitting a bucket of balls on the range. That seemed very manageable.

During our early years in Waccabuc, I played at other nearby courses, but not that often. When Greg visited, we'd play some of the courses near our house, like Pehquenakonck Country Club and the Salem Golf Club. While Waccabuc Country Club had a waitlist, you could join the Salem Golf Club by paying a small initiation fee. At that point, I really didn't understand how golf worked. I would go to the range a little bit. I would sometimes play golf with a friend. I was still using Greg's clubs then. Marcela wasn't golfing too much with me. We hadn't yet fully immersed ourselves in golf.

We were also pretty busy. Our son, Matthew, was six, starting first grade. Isabella was in nursery school. They had all sorts of activities going on. Professionally, Marcela and I were also building our careers. Marcela was running campaigns to help presidents in Latin America get democratically elected. I had been traveling internationally nearly every week.

Even with my busy schedule, I was gradually getting the golf bug. I was practicing a little bit more at Salem Golf Club, and my friend William was a member at the Waccabuc Country Club. In 2000, Marcela and I finally decided we'd try to join the Waccabuc Country Club. William advised that the best way was to become active in the community of Waccabuc and get to know our neighbors. At that point we were mostly meeting people through the elementary and nursery school that our kids attended. We needed to branch out.

William graciously introduced us to some people who lived in Waccabuc and were also members of the club. One of our neighbors down the road was a woman named Susan Henry. She was a descendant of the Mead family of Brooklyn that had originally created the hamlet of Waccabuc. Susan was a strong land preservationist and an active member in the Westchester Land Trust. She was very committed to preserving open space, and that was one of our most important issues as well. We told Susan we wanted to get involved in the community. Susan and her husband, Jim, a delightful storyteller, lived in a landmarked house at the top of our block. Susan was all business with an amazing soft side once she got to know you.

I was working for Hillary Clinton at the time—it was the year she got elected to the Senate. My company had also represented Bill Clinton, and Susan very quickly caught on that Marcela and I had political know-how. She told me about a bond referendum to preserve open land in the town of Lewisboro that would be on the ballot in November 2000. "Can you help us?" she asked, and I told her it happened to be right up our alley. I made some suggestions about what a campaign would look like. She was delighted. I also did a poll and found that the number one priority for people was to keep the town beautiful and natural, and to reject commercial development.

Still, we had to get people to vote. I knew that the 2000 turnout would be high in the town. It was a presidential year. It was an open seat. Bill Clinton had had an amazing eight years as president, but it would be a tight race between Al Gore and George H. W. Bush. So, I designed some direct mail that we sent out to all the people in the town of Lewisboro. We did some robocalls. Susan had the idea that we should present the results to the town council. Suddenly I was involved in a very tight battle over the bond issue in our local town of Lewisboro.

Long story short, we won the land bond, and it's been one of the most wonderful things that we did. We met so many people that summer and immersed ourselves in the community. So, in the quest to be more involved in the country club and be able to play golf with my family, I found myself involved in town politics. I'd always advise people to know who's on both sides of the aisle before you take sides. I wouldn't have done anything different, but the political scene delayed our gratification a bit. Let's just say, the issue was heated and conflict arose. Our application went on hold, and we didn't get into the Waccabuc Country Club until 2003. Sometimes it's not easy to belong. But in the end, it was all worth it.

At this point in my life, I probably felt like many of you reading this book. I didn't know much about country club life apart from what I'd seen in movies like *Caddyshack*. My father used to say, "Why would anyone join a country club when we pay so much in taxes for all of these beautiful parks?" He would point out Waveland tennis courts, which were public. Oak Street Beach was right in front of my house, and the Lake Shore golf course was just down Lake Shore Drive. Dad didn't want me to pay for more and then limit my choices. So, no country clubs. Marcela grew up with some friends at the Jockey Club in Buenos Aires, but what bonded Jorge Sixto Miguel (her father in Buenos Aires) and Howard Berland (my father in Chicago) is that they were decidedly anti–country club.

I guess Marcela and I just figured it out for ourselves.

PRACTICE, PRACTICE, PRACTICE

I was serious about getting my act together, so I started taking lessons with a golf pro at the Waccabuc Country Club named John McPhee. My session was at eight o'clock in the morning. I called it "Breakfast with McPhee." We'd play nine holes (the front or the back. It was always an issue if it was ladies' day, because men were not allowed on the course before noon, but John always had a work-around). He'd give me a stroke per hole, and if I ever beat him, the lesson was free. Over the course of five years, I never beat John McPhee once. I probably never had a chance. John holds the course record at Waccabuc to this day and played in the U.S. Senior Open in 2002 and finished T-61. He is pretty good!

To say that John was an old-school, cantankerous person would make him sound more pleasant than he was. But he was incredibly lovable and patient with me, and I looked forward to my lessons all week long. Often, I could see the sheer frustration in his face as I would hit a shot, or I would swing the club and see in his face that he had never seen someone hit the shot as badly as I hit it. I'll never forget the look of utter bewilderment. Like my mother, he would call me Michael. "Michael, that's just not going to work. Why are you twirling the club at the top of your swing?" But then, with remarkable patience and a steady hand, he'd show me what I did wrong and how to improve. I'd had teachers and mentors in my life, but I'd never had a relationship quite like the one I had with John McPhee. The last time I saw John was when I played in a pro–am in Palm Springs, California. John came to watch William and me tee off. As soon as I hit my shot, he screamed, "You have gotten a lot better since I had you!" The ultimate compliment from John.

Jeff Smith, currently the director of instruction at the Vintage Club in Indian Wells, California and Pine Canyon in Flagstaff, Arizona, became a mentor and teacher of mine when he was the director of instruction at Eagle Springs Golf Club in Wolcott, Colorado, and I spent time with him during our family visits there. Jeff is also the co-host of the nationally syndicated radio show *Those Weekend Golf Guys*, an easygoing, fun, and accessible program for regular golfers like me. On the show, Jeff and his co-host John Ashton will cover every golf topic on your mind, I promise you.

I can't count the number of times I've picked Jeff's brain to find ways to improve my game. He gave me the "five keys to a golf swing." Here they are:

1. Aim the club at your target.

2. Square the club face. Make it face the target at impact.

3. Swing the club face to the same spot each time.

4. Release the club and understand the physics: The club must get below the ball to get it up/learn how to go fast.

5. Swing smoothly and easily and learn to love the extra distance.

As I look back at them now, they seem so obvious, but they weren't obvious to me for the first twenty years that I took golf lessons, and they only made sense once I knew them. I often wonder if golf would have been easier had I started with this approach. In most of my work as a consultant, we tell our clients that they spend too much time telling their consumers what they do, but they don't ever explain the "how" or the "why." People can't trust you if they only know the "what." Most people I was taking lessons from were trying to show me what to do—often taking videos of me and comparing them to other golfers. But I'm not a visual learner. I am a pollster. I read and analyze data. I learn by hearing and analyzing and then drawing conclusions. In that spirit, Jeff's five keys were right in my wheelhouse. Thanks, Jeff. I never take a swing when I'm not thinking about these keys.

LEARNING TO BELONG

I played my first tournament at Waccabuc Country Club in 2004. They had an annual, three-day, member-guest tournament where a member could invite someone from another club to play in a two-person team.

My friend William had been playing in this tournament for many years with his friend Sam. William and Sam went all the way back to lower school. I also knew Sam because he was in my YPO chapter.

The three-day, member-guest tournament was always a fun weekend for me, even before I played in it and before I was a member of the Waccabuc Country Club, because William made it so much fun. During the tournament, William's house was the center of the action with families and friends around all weekend. It would culminate in a party on Saturday night for all William's friends and neighbors—golfers and nongolfers.

At dinner William and Sam would engage in golf banter. I would listen and smile, although early on I had no idea what they were talking about. One night when William said to Sam, "You have hands of steel when you putt," I had no idea what he meant. I realized I didn't want to be in the position of not knowing anymore. I wanted to learn not just the moves but the language. And I did.

Back to the Waccabuc three-day tournament. I invited my YPO friend Tony, who was also William's friend, to be my guest. As I mentioned earlier, our friendship and golf partnership would become one of the enduring pleasures of my life. Tony was like the big brother I never had. He is tough, demanding, and loyal. Tony taught me the ins and outs of how to play tournament golf, the patience that's required to focus on each and every shot, the dynamics that happen within a team and against an opponent, and the good-natured psychological warfare that goes on at a golf tournament. As Marcela says, nobody enters a tournament to lose. Tony is relentless and demands full commitment. He expects and gets full effort at all times. I didn't (and probably still don't) have that kind of discipline. Tony showed me what it takes to win.

That first year we ended up in the middle of the pack. Not great, but not terrible. The second year we won our flight, which means that we came first in our division, which was a boost, but we lost in the shootout. The shootout is when the winners of each flight (there were twelve flights total) played in a single elimination hole. All twelve teams would tee off on the tenth tee box and then play alternate shots. The winner was the team that finished the hole with the fewest shots. If there was a tie, they'd play the eleventh hole and keep going until one of them won.

Playing in the shootout at the Waccabuc three-day member-guest tournament is like playing in a PGA tournament, with hundreds of Waccabuc players, their guests, and their families watching and driving in golf carts with their favorite adult beverages on the tenth fairway. It is loud. It is fun. It is nerve-racking for a golfer like me.

To start the shootout, they call the name of the winning team, and the team has to decide which golfer will tee off. William and Sam had made it to the shootout many times but had never won. I really didn't think it was possible to win the shootout—so many good shots were required, in front of a huge gallery. It seemed like a lot of pressure to me. Even if I was partnered with a lower-handicapped partner, I would have to hit at least two of the shots. In front of all those people. No way.

Playing in the Waccabuc three-day, member-guest tournament became an annual event for Tony and me. Despite the extreme heat and humidity, we were having fun, and we were also having success. Our third year in the tournament was exciting. We were on a roll. We were beating all the teams we were playing, and we won our flight by a wide margin. We had made the shootout, and it felt different. Tony was confident. William and Sam were there in a cart, rooting for us and giving us advice. We decided that Tony would hit the tee shot. He hit a beautiful shot that unfortunately veered a little bit to the left and went into the sand trap. I realized that I was going to have to hit the next shot out of the bunker.

I was extremely nervous. I was conscious of being in the spotlight, and I didn't know if I could do it. Then, to make matters much worse, my nose started bleeding, which can happen when I get nervous. The timing could not have been more inconvenient and embarrassing. Blood was dripping out of my nose as I stepped into the bunker. Eyes wide, Tony handed me a napkin, and I wadded it and stuck it up my nostrils, looking ridiculous but stopping the blood flow.

The whole crowd at Waccabuc was watching. William and Sam were in their cart being positive and giving me advice on where to hit my shot (as if I had any control), and Tony was calm, talking me through it step by step as he always does, and reminding me to breathe. I looked at the ball, and I swung, and somehow the ball came perfectly out of the bunker and landed on the fairway. We moved on to the third shot, and Tony hit another beauty. Then I, with the napkin still hanging out of my nose, hit another good shot to keep us in contention. It was a three-quarter, 9-iron shot that McPhee had taught me only a few days before the tournament, and it worked! It was a surreal moment. Our ball was on the green with Tony in position to make a putt.

There was more pressure than ever, because now the whole club was *really* watching us. It was a magical moment, even though my nose was bleeding, and I was a little lightheaded. Everything went our way. Long story short, Tony took an aggressive line (which he always does) and made the putt—and we won!

Plenty of people came up to congratulate us, but I didn't really know many of them. I didn't have a friend network at the club yet. A member-guest team has magic when people know the winners. We were the outsiders. I was determined to change that. I made it a point to get more involved.

It became for me a great lesson of how social golf is played. I understood that success in a tournament required a number of skills—golf strategy, chemistry with a partner, the ability to focus. What nobody tells you is that belonging isn't automatic. You have to earn it over time.

Maybe the most valuable lesson I learned was the impact that a golf partnership could have on me. Tony and I had such chemistry, and being with him helped me focus, even when my nose was spurting blood. But most important, my friendship with Tony became one of the most enduring and important relationships of my life. We were friends, and we were golf partners, which involved another level of understanding and commitment. Tony has skills like no other. He can detect changes in my breathing and know what I am thinking. That doesn't come from going to dinner together or hanging out sometimes. That comes from golfing.

Nearly twenty years later, I still play in the Waccabuc member-guest. My latest partner, until my grandson can play with me, is my best friend from high school, Nat. Like me growing up in Chicago, he took up golf when he was an adult. Nat is a headmaster at a great school in Racine, Wisconsin, and has some flexibility in the summer so he comes to Waccabuc and spends the weekend with me. I am not sure whether we have more fun on the golf course or at home, but it is a great time. Nat likes to win, which keeps the pressure on me.

I wonder what my golf skills are. I know that my skill on the golf course is that I don't let people get stuck on an outcome or a result. I keep it positive and live for the next shot. I know who I am playing with—some people like to talk a lot, some people like to have small wagers and play games, and some people don't even like to keep score. They just want to be in the moment.

If I never had to fill out a golf scorecard again, I don't think I would miss it. I do always keep score and submit my score because that is the norm to maintain a handicap. I am not sure it does a lot for me personally. I don't get upset when I score high, and I don't get too excited if I shoot a low score. I know it always reverts.

Actually, the best use I ever found for a scorecard was when I was playing with Gary Briggs. Gary is a brilliant guy who has had a hand in some of the groundbreaking business ventures of our time, including McKinsey, IBM, Pepsi, eBay, Pay Pal, Google, and Facebook. Gary is one of those people who makes a difference every time he opens his mouth.

I'd gotten to know Gary when he was CMO of Facebook, and I was doing work for the company. Of course, we played golf together. One day we were out on the golf course, and I was describing my newest venture, tracking momentum. Always a fast thinker, Gary immediately had insights. He looked around for something to write on and found only a golf scorecard. He pulled it out and scribbled his thoughts, which were so on the money I included them in my book *Maximum Momentum*. I still have that scorecard, and consider Gary's notes the best scorecard use ever.

THE POWER OF CONNECTIVITY

Keith Ward is a consummate networker, and his credits as a banker and a wealth advisor at J.P. Morgan are impressive. But when I talk to him about golf, I feel that I'm seeing the real Keith—the person without titles or glamor or the trappings of success.

In his early career years, Keith wasn't a regular golfer. He got new clubs on his wedding day, but he didn't play much. But after his divorce, he began to play more. "There were some lonely days," he recalled. "I was getting used to not having my boys on a consistent basis, just midweek visits and every other weekend. I had a lot of time on my hands, and I started hanging out with some guys who liked to golf on the weekends. I didn't have a club, and we'd use local courses. I was a big user of Pound Ridge Golf Club. And I really started to get the bug. In fact, I got the bug so much so that when I met my second wife, Maria, some six years later, she looked in my closet and asked if I was a golf pro."

For Keith, making connections and helping others is the greatest value of golf. The importance of connections is something that was instilled in him from childhood. "My dad was a house painter. We didn't have a lot," he said. "But he always talked about the power of connectivity. He used to tell me: 'Your network is your net worth, and it takes a long time to develop that network. And it's very easy, in a short amount of time, to completely blow that network up right with how you behave.' He'd give me those lessons, and he'd push me to expand my network. So did my mother, in her own way. She was incredibly out-going. She loved helping people, and she was very authentic. Between my parents, I learned to value making connections, and when I began to golf seriously, I found my people."

PLAYING "HOST GOLF"

"Golfing with new people for the first time is like a blind date. You just don't know how it is going to go until you get there and start golfing." I laughed when my new partner made this observation. It was so true. I was being hosted at a golf course that I have wanted to play for the past ten years. My host was a friend's brother, who was a member, along with one of his friends who were also strangers to me.

I approached my "blind date" a little nervous. I had no idea how the game would play out. What was going to happen? On the third hole, I had a terrifying downhill chip with a flag very close. Either I was going to hit a great chip that spun and stopped, or my ball was going off the green. Instead, I hit the shot nearly perfectly. My ball landed soft and spun just behind my host's ball mark, which meant I would putt first, and he would be able to see the way the putt broke. Good for him. He asked me if he needed to move his mark. I said: "It isn't in my way. I can putt over it"—which I did. I missed my putt by just a little bit. He had the same putt, made it, and had his first par of the day.

Afterward he said to me, "You are playing perfect 'host golf.'" I'd never heard the term, but I instantly knew what it meant. I had lined up his putt, and he made it. It was my pleasure. The rest of the round was great, and we'll play again soon. We are golf buddies now.

BROADENING MY GOLF HORIZONS

I'm always pushing my boundaries and trying to get better at golf. That's how I happened to be taking golf lessons in Uruguay after the pandemic. What was I doing in Uruguay?

Marcela was born and raised in Buenos Aires, Argentina. During her summers, her family spent a month or so each year in Punta del Este, Uruguay. Growing up in Chicago, I don't think I could have even conceived that a place like Punta del Este existed other than in the movies. First of all, geographically it is south of Brazil and east of Buenos Aires. As the name implies, it is a point that juts out into the Atlantic Ocean. It is an endless surfer beach with big waves, a nice breeze, and plenty of large Miami-Beach-style buildings. As you get farther out, it turns into single family homes and has spectacular villages like Faro José Ignacio. Punta del Este is for tourists, mostly from Argentina, Brazil, and of course Uruguay.

The pandemic taught us that we didn't have to be limited to one location or another, especially since our kids have left the nest. We could work from anywhere. So, Marcela decided to look for other places we could live part-time. I only had a few criteria: 1) There had to be a golf course. 2) There had to be a beachfront. 3) There had to be easy access back to the states. 4) The food had to be great.

Punta del Este was popular, and Marcela still had lots of friends there, so she started looking at properties. A few years before we bought anything, I went down with Isabella to check it out. I loved it immediately. As a throwaway, I told Marcela, "If I ever sell my business, I will buy the apartment that you choose as a gift." At that time, I had no intention of selling my business, so while it was a nice gesture, I didn't think it had much of a chance of coming true.

Then 2022 came along and I sold my business. I kept my promise and bought a property in Punta del Este. We joined La Barra Golf Club in Punta del Este. And now I live in Uruguay a few months each year.

We have made so many wonderful friends there that by the beginning of October, I am getting ready for our second summer.

The culture of Argentina and Uruguay is more direct than in the United States. After a few rounds at La Barra, my new friends Daniel and Claudio told me that I needed to take some lessons. Daniel and Claudio are beautiful golfers with nearly perfect form. If they knew how many lessons I had taken, they would be shocked. But they were right.

During that first season in Punta, I decided to finally deal with parts of my golf swing that were inconsistent. I'd always played golf to enjoy the social and networking aspects. My score was never the important part. I wanted to play well so I could focus on the enjoyment of it.

But now I had some time to finally practice. I made the decision to play more consistently and eliminate the volatility in my swing. I had been working on it for years with various pros. They had each taken me along the journey and allowed me to enjoy twenty-plus years of golf. But now it was time to get serious.

The best instructor in Punta was a pro named Max who didn't speak any English. My Spanish is just okay. I can manage the grocery store, can get around a menu at a restaurant, and can be polite in an elevator, but I certainly didn't have the technical vocabulary for a golf lesson.

On the other hand, I thought I should give it a try. In a flash of self-awareness, I thought, maybe my gregarious nature was getting in the way of learning. Maybe I talk too much to the instructor, and the language barrier would help me focus on the actual game. Without the chitchat, maybe I'd get serious. And Max could instruct me with his movements, his eyes, and the sensations that I feel in the clubs and the little Spanish that I could actually understand.

It was a fascinating experience. Taking lessons with Max in broken Spanish was like analyzing a poll. I could tell the parts of the lessons that were important and having an impact on my outcome. I could ask a question, get his response, and then try it.

Where is it written
that you have to conform?

—STEPHEN MALBON,
Malbon Golf

And then he suggested something magical—a change in my grip.

The easiest fix in my golf swing turned out to be the most impactful—I changed my grip. Seems simple, but it had eluded me until then. Changing the grip also allowed a flow in my swing as I felt the club going over my back. And I could now take a full turn with the club head going through the ball and straight to the target. It was a sensation I'd never felt before. Suddenly the ball was going in the direction that I aimed at, and I was swinging through lighter than I ever had. *Wow.* I was elated. I couldn't believe I was actually improving my swing at long last.

Somehow, I felt it was more than that. Yes, I changed my swing, but I was also starting to close on writer Malcolm Gladwell's idea of ten thousand hours of practice—that is, if you practice something correctly for ten thousand hours, you will develop expertise. I am in no way implying that it was the right ten thousand hours, but I had been working hard at golf. Golf was not casual for me. It had become a glue that was holding many parts of my life together.

During my time in Punta del Este, I received a text from William. Would I like to join him as an amateur player at the pro-am American Express PGA Golf Tournament in Palm Springs in mid-January 2023? This was a three-day PGA tournament with a practice day. I said yes, realizing that it was a big moment. I would be playing in my first pro-am tournament, and I hoped I was ready.

7

THE GODS WERE SMILING

Sometimes golfers will talk about golf gods as in "Don't anger the golf gods." Well, if there are golf gods, I think they sent me an angel when I played my first PGA pro-am tournament. In pro-ams, professional golfers play with amateurs—typically, one professional to three amateurs. The amateurs get the experience of playing with a pro and briefly blur the line between professionals and amateurs. It's rare for this to happen in a sport, but pro golfers usually go along because it's part of their sponsorship deals. It's a good way for sponsors to get maximum benefit. They can entertain their clients. The pro-ams will typically happen on the Tuesday before a pro tournament, played Thursday to Saturday.

The American Express (previously known by many names, including the Bob Hope Desert Classic) is different. It's a PGA pro-am tournament played Thursday to Saturday, and in this format, each amateur is paired with a different PGA tour professional.

Remember, my objective in playing golf was to be with my friends, meet new friends, and have fun, so I'd never been interested in a professional golf tournament or thought that I was qualified to play in a professional tournament. But the American Express was serious business—three days of amateurs being paired with three different professionals on three different golf courses in PGA West, which is composed of a total of six courses in Palm Springs.

I hadn't been to Palm Springs since I was seventeen years old—thirty-eight years earlier. The idea of playing in a professional setting in front of a crowd didn't scare me. I had given plenty of speeches. I had made many live TV appearances. But playing in a PGA tournament? That wasn't really my thing. First, I wasn't sure my golf game was up to the challenge. Yet, when the opportunity came, I didn't hesitate. In my book *Maximum Momentum*, I wrote about the common assumption that some people are just lucky and some aren't. It's not true. What *is* true is that some people take advantage of opportunities and others don't. I hadn't been looking for this opportunity, but I knew I had to take it.

I looked at it, and I said, of course, I want to play in a professional-amateur tournament. Of course, I want to play for three days with PGA professionals, PGA caddies, rope lines keeping the fans behind them. Of course, I want to go to Palm Springs, because in a way it's the biggest opportunity that anybody who is as passionate about golf as I am could get.

Playing in a PGA tournament was a different experience than playing at the Augusta National Golf Course. At Augusta, the location was steeped in tradition. For the American Express, I was going to play golf with the best golf professionals in the world. Remember, I am a data guy. I was going to see firsthand PGA tour professionals, their fans, and how the pros interact with their fans.

I had nine weeks to prepare, and I played almost every day. I prepared my swing, but mostly I prepared my mind to get in the zone of caring about my score and taking the game seriously at a higher level. After all the years of just playing good enough to keep the ball ahead of me, I knew that wouldn't be enough. The point of a PGA event is to compete and to win. I wasn't thinking that this was social at all. It was about winning.

When we arrived in Palm Springs, the golf gods sent me an angel, and his name was David O'Donovan. David was the PGA caddie who would shepherd me through this incredible program experience.

A caddie can be like having a thought partner at work—someone you can bounce ideas off of, and who will help boost your confidence. That was David. We played a practice session together at PGA West, one of the two Nicklaus courses. David helped me make better decisions and gave me the reinforcement I needed. And, like an angel, when he was there miracles started to happen with my golf.

This was a first for me! My swing was smooth, the ball went where I wanted it to go, my intended shots just worked. Miraculously, David saw and understood me—the man who loved playing with his friends and loved the game. In his presence, everything else faded away. The crowds disappeared, the water hazards disappeared, the bunkers disappeared. I was just playing pure golf. I couldn't believe it. All that hard work and effort to slow my swing down, to square my club face, to follow through all my distances was working. And I thought, *After twenty-some years of golf, it came together.*

Playing in a golf tournament at the PGA level is unlike any time I've ever played golf with my friends, with my wife, or with my son. And yet, it was just like every time I ever played golf with my friends, with my wife, or with my son—except for the phenomenal result.

I started wondering about the difference, and I realized that it was simple. I was just having fun. I was fully enjoying the best parts of golf, and the thrill of being part of something so magical that I've done casually for so long.

Playing with a partner in a best ball format, which means it's my best ball or my partner's best ball, is not new for me. I've played many tournaments with my friends and my son and my wife. But this time I played one of my best rounds ever. I think it was a result of being in that environment where I could experience the true joy of the ball going up, the ball coming down, and the ball going into the hole. That was different than my normal golf game, because at the PGA tournament there were a lot of people keeping their eyes on your ball. When I played with my friends or even in regular tournaments, I always had to find my ball. And I had a tendency to spray the ball (I do so less now) and the ball could go anywhere, and I had to find it. At the American Express, I just had to hit!

The Amex experience reaffirmed everything I ever thought about golf, which is that it's just fun. And I started to explain the concept of this book to the golf professionals I was playing with. I asked them, "What if golf was just fun? What if it was a great way to spend time with your friends and family, to spend time with your wife, to spend time with your kids, and not keep score?" They were dumbfounded by the whole idea that golf could just be fun because this is how they make a living. I totally get that. But for the other 99 percent of us, we just do it for enjoyment. And that day, with the gods of golf smiling on me, I really felt it.

8

THE BEST FRIENDSHIPS
ARE GOLF FRIENDSHIPS

I've played golf in Asia, I've played golf in Europe, I've played golf in South America, I've played golf in North America, I've played golf in Australia, I've played in Africa. No matter where I am, the one thing I do is play golf and meet new people. I have built friendships based on golf all over the world. There are subtle differences in some of the customs and some of the habits of golf, which make golf fantastic. But everything else is the same. There is global common ground in golf.

I've gone on a couple of golf trips with the previously mentioned Young Presidents Organization. I have always enjoyed playing as part of the YPO. Golf was the excuse, but it's really the adventure of playing and meeting new people. The YPO golf network has made connections for me in so many places. One year I played the Ocean Course in Kiawah, South Carolina, where Phil Mickelson won the PGA Championship at fifty years and eleven months old, becoming the oldest man to win a major. I played on the same Ocean Course that he won the tournament on.

My golf friends and I have traveled to courses from Bandon Dunes in Oregon to Pebble Beach in Carmel, California. The games we played there were important, but the most important part for me was the people we were with, the time that we had, and the events that happened afterward. While clients can come and go, golf friendships endure.

YPO has a dual structure—there is international membership that is comprised of local chapters. Within the chapters, there are smaller groups called forums. A forum has eight to ten members, and my forum met ten times a year for twenty years. We held all our meetings in New York City, and once a year we would go away for two days for an off-site that included a facilitator.

Luckily, our entire forum was golf obsessed. Each year we went off-site to a place that had great golf. We went to Pinehurst, the Greenbrier, Atlantic City Country Club, the Breakers, East Hampton Golf Club, the New Albany Country Club, Streamsong, Sea Island, Century Country Club, and GlenArbor Golf Club. The purpose of the off-site was personal growth. The side benefit was the time that we spent on the golf course—sharing ideas, catching up, and creating relationships that extended beyond YPO.

THE DUBAI EXPERIENCE

In 2004 I went on the YPO trip to Dubai, which was called the YPO Golf World Championship. I had been to Dubai many times early in my career. I never thought I could be invited to a golf world championship because I didn't think I was of that caliber. I am a 20-plus handicapper. But I thought it would be a lot of fun to play golf in Dubai. So, I signed up. And there I met a number of interesting characters from all over the world who had come to Dubai to play golf.

I went with Sam (another 20-plus handicapper). We were paired up, and we really enjoyed playing. It wasn't a strict PGA tournament. We were playing different courses in Dubai, in different formats. I made some great friends in one day. I played in a foursome with a guy named

Khashoggi. Sam and I thought, *well, that's an interesting name.* So, Sam asked him, "What do you do?"

Then I remembered: Khashoggi was the name of an arms dealer. I thought, *Only in YPO can you meet people like this.* Later, I'd shudder at the thought that I'd been playing with a notorious Middle East arms dealer. But this was the early days in Dubai, and Khashoggi wasn't well known—just a typical guy playing golf. (This reference is to Adnan Khashoggi, not the journalist Jamal Khashoggi, who was tragically assassinated in 2018.)

My first trip to Dubai had been in 1993. At that time, Dubai consisted of a few major roads, some buildings, and an incredible master plan. I was doing consumer market research for an oil company named EPPCO. In many developing countries, the first part of building the infrastructure is to understand where the service stations will go, and then building accordingly. So, I saw Dubai just as it was starting.

Dubai is made up of four groups—Emirati (the Dubai Nationals), the Western Expats (from Europe, North America, and Australia), South Asians, and Arabs from various countries in the Middle East and North Africa. In 2001, I was working on a political project for Sheik Mohamed's office. The objective was to find ways of creating more social equality in the United Arab Emirates. As their society was coming together, it was very important that each group felt represented. I had been working on the project all summer, and the final presentation was scheduled for September 13 in Dubai.

At the same time, I was working locally in New York for Mike Bloomberg, who was running for mayor in New York City as a Republican. Primary day was September 11, 2001. It was going to be a busy week for me. Our polling showed that Bloomberg would win quite handily, so that was going to be a fun celebration. The real election would come in the November general election, either against Fernando Ferrer, a Democrat who was running a historical campaign to be the first Hispanic mayor of New York, or Mark Green, a Democrat and perennial candidate.

My plan was to go to Mike's victory party and then leave for Dubai the next day.

There was no victory party, and there was no trip to Dubai. September 11 changed everything. Mike won the mayor's race in November, defeating Mark Green and telling New Yorkers that the city needed a businessman, not a politician. Mike was also endorsed by then "America's Mayor" Rudy Giuliani. Funny how people change over time.

Mike went on to serve three terms as New York's mayor. Bloomberg Philanthropies, which he started after he left office, is one of the most impactful organizations in the world.

My trip to Dubai on September 12 was canceled and turned into a video call. In those days, video calls were done in dedicated facilities that had special equipment and high-speed hookups. I always wondered if the FBI was listening to my presentation that day. If they were, they would have heard the social blueprint for the Emirate that is the modern Dubai.

So, it should be no surprise that when I had the opportunity in 2004 to play in the YPO World Championship, I took it. I hadn't been back to Dubai since I'd done the project. I was curious to see how Dubai had come together. Were the plans being implemented? Did the hotels get constructed? When I visited in the nineties, there were only one or two golf courses. Now, I knew, there were many. The most famous was the Emirates Golf Club, which hosted the Dubai Desert Classic. It was the first grass golf course in the Middle East when it opened in 1988. And it was one of three courses we played while we were there.

I didn't recognize Dubai when I arrived. The luxury buildings that Dubai is famous for had been built. We stayed at a hotel that had luxury suites in bungalow-like buildings with our own butler. To get from bungalow to bungalow, we took a boat. It reminded me of being in Venice.

Dubai was just becoming a tourist destination. I was struck by the pool system. They pumped in cold water to cool them down. Coming from Chicago where the water started cold and was rarely heated, this was new to me.

In the middle of the second round, we were playing a sand course that lived up to its reputation when a huge sandstorm came up. Suddenly we were forced to seek cover as the wind whipped around us, and we couldn't see one foot ahead.

A TASMANIAN ADVENTURE

As I was writing this book, I decided that I would go on another golf trip with YPO, whose golf network connects with golfers all over the world. This golf tournament was in Tasmania, Australia. Funny thing, I even had a connection there.

I'd lived in Sydney, Australia, in 1993, during the earliest part of my career. In fact, I deliberately set things up so I could live there. Maybe I just needed to get away from the cramped world of New York City. Maybe I wanted to flex my muscles and be independent. I grabbed at the chance.

Our firm had an opportunity to write a contract for an oil company named Caltex, which was a joint venture between Texaco and Chevron that operated in countries east of the Suez Canal. The study was an international brand reimaging and reputation study for Caltex, before their large capital investment to upgrade all their service stations and build convenience stores. Its main markets were China, Singapore, Thailand, the Philippines, Australia, and New Zealand. They were going to run the project out of Sydney, Australia. So, as a twenty-four-year-old, I wrote my job description into the proposal as the on-site project manager, which meant I'd be living in Sydney for the duration.

Now I had two opportunities. One, I'd travel to and live in a place on the other side of the world; and two, it would give my career the space and distance I thought it needed for a momentum boost. Even at that young age, I didn't want to always be in the position of number two. I wanted to be number one. By writing myself into the proposal to live in Sydney, I would have a level of autonomy just with the time zones and the requirements of the team. I would have my own operation, my own research, and I would be more embedded in the team. I'd be a twentysomething project manager of a seven-figure research project. It doesn't get much better than that.

After that experience, I'd been back to Australia once in 2000 and a second time with my son in 2014 for his eighteenth birthday. Now, with a golf trip to Tasmania, I decided to take Marcela and Isabella.

If you think about it, Tasmania might be the single farthest point from New York. It was as far as I could possibly go to play golf. I was eager to experience a new place so far away. So, I signed up.

Marcela and I left on February 5, 2024, from Vail to Denver to Los Angeles, where we met our daughter, Isabella. From there we all flew to Sydney. For the first couple days, we went sightseeing. We went to Bondi Beach and Manly Beach. We saw the Sydney Opera House, had a delicious dinner at the Apollo restaurant, and visited the neighborhood of Kings Cross. Then I was off to Tasmania to play golf. I'd be going to Launceston, a city in northern Tasmania that I couldn't really pronounce, playing at a beautiful destination golf course called Barnbougle Dunes.

On the flight from Sydney to Launceston, I met Piers, who was the organizer of the trip. Piers worked at a legendary club called the New South Wales Club. After we picked up luggage and loaded it into the car for our hour drive to Barnbougle Dunes, Piers did his best imitation of Crocodile Dundee. If you recall, Crocodile Dundee was sort of a swashbuckling, larger-than-life character from Australia. Piers wasn't trying, and maybe I am stereotyping him, but I promise you I felt like I was in a movie. Piers regaled us with stories about the snakes in Tasmania—the browns, the Red Belly blacks, the Tigers. I started to feel a little nervous. Then he told a story about Steve Irwin, a famous Australian who wrestled crocodiles and ultimately was killed by a stingray who stung him straight in the heart while he was swimming.

I was beginning to sweat. This was a destination golfing trip, and I was hearing about deadly snakes and crocodiles. What kind of destination was this?

Piers mentioned that his secret passion was wrestling and capturing snakes. He described all the people he knew who had been bitten by snakes. I happen to be afraid of snakes, and the idea of wrestling them is beyond my imagination. I told Piers that, and he replied in a solemn voice, something I'll never forget: "Fear is good, mate. It'll keep you alive." What the hell?

By the time we got to the course, I could see that there was a pretty good storm coming in. But Australians are very hardy people. A little bad weather is not going to keep them off the course. I coincidentally was traveling with Craig, a fellow YPO player from Toronto, Canada. Craig and I knew each other from a previous YPO trip that we had taken to Egypt earlier in the year. We watched as the storm was blowing in and the lightning flashing over the horizon, but the organizers were calling, "Let's tee off." The show was going to go on. (As an aside, golfers are obsessed with weather. We can give any weather reporters a run for their money and always have a POV of what is going to happen.)

I teed off and hit a great shot right into the fairway. My next shot was good. And then I started getting bombarded by bugs flying into my face as the rain got closer. Back in the pro shop, I'd asked for suntan lotion and was told: "Look, mate, you're not going to need suntan lotion today. Maybe an umbrella." Now I wished I'd also picked up some bug spray.

Then off in the distance I saw lightning. No golfer likes lightning! I asked nervously, "Do you have lightning detectors?" Most courses in the United States, Canada, and Europe do. And I was told, "Look, mate, you're much more likely to get nicked by a snake than you are to be struck by lightning." That was supposed to be comforting?

Craig and I made it through one and a half holes before we decided we were going back.

But there was no culture of "going back" once you started a game. And there was no warning system for the lightning. As I watched the streaks of lightning, I flashed on a scene from *Caddyshack* when the priest gets struck by lightning while having the best round of his life. I was playing a really good game myself.

Then Craig said, "I'm long past having to impress the coach." I heard what he was saying—basically, that there was no reason to play in the rain and lightning in Barnbougle Dunes to impress anyone. Such words of wisdom! We were comfortable enough with each other and knew we had nothing to prove to each other.

Just then Piers, who was poking at the grass with his 7-iron, called us over. I could tell by the excitement on his face that he'd found a snake and was trying to capture it to show me. "Fear is good. It'll keep you safe," I said, and joined my partners walking off the course.

A BONDING EXPERIENCE

The YPO golf trip to Barnbougle Dunes really demonstrated the value of networking. The outsider might think the YPO golf network was a network of great golfers, but that wasn't necessarily the case. Being in a golf network means that you understand what it is to meet different people from all over the world. And you understand that golf is a great common denominator. Golf brings people together. In the YPO golf network, people came to Tasmania from Toronto, Washington, DC, Tulsa, New York, Melbourne, Sydney, Brisbane, Calgary—from all over the world. We came for the same reason, to be with other golfers. In fact, most of us weren't great golfers. But we were great networkers. We were people who loved to travel to meet new people and enjoy new settings and experiences while we golfed.

The first night we were joined by a pro golfer who gave us some golf tips. It was mildly interesting, but not why we were there. The second night we heard from the guy who developed Barnbougle Dunes, and he told us the backstory of why he developed it, the process he went through, and how he managed it. That was much more interesting to us. We were intrigued by the backstory of how he took a very average farm in Tasmania, Australia, and turned it into a top ten destination golf course. For us YPO folks, that was a conversation that could have gone on all night.

The next day we were up bright and early and back on the course. Not a cloud in the sky. My golf game on this trip was pretty good. But to be honest, the last thing I was thinking about was my golf game. I was mostly thinking about the great people I was meeting (and the snakes in the rough). That day I was playing in a foursome with some terrific guys from Canada, and we spent a lot of time talking about our lives and businesses and were really getting to know one another. These were people I would definitely be connecting with once we got home—we all understood the power of networking.

I met a great guy from Brisbane, Australia, and we got to know each other. He had a fascinating credit business. I met someone from the Gold Coast in Australia who was integrating golf into his senior developments. In fact, he was coming to the United States a few weeks after our trip to meet with the top range developers in Houston and Orlando. So, now I have a network in Australia. I can go play the New South Wales Club golf course in Sydney, or I can play Royal Melbourne—the top golf courses. The remoteness of the venues makes them highly desirable places to golf. People enjoy being off the grid.

When you're in a remote location, you might play eighteen or thirty-six holes of golf. But even if you play eight to ten hours a day, that still leaves fourteen hours. Then what do you do? In a remote place like Tasmania there's nothing to do but enjoy the company of your fellow golfers. It's a unique bonding experience.

It takes a big effort to get to Tasmania, but it pays off in the relationships, which have a lasting impact. Twenty-six hours on a plane to Australia is a down payment on future adventures.

I am so thankful to Andy Winces for helping to put the trip together. Everything in YPO is volunteer. Andy was herding YPOers from all over the world. No easy task, but he made it look easy. The Aussie way.

When Craig and I were bonding, he started telling me about his favorite home course at Lake Muskoka, which is two hours north of Toronto, deep in the woods. I'd been going to Toronto for most of my career, starting with my work in Waterloo with BlackBerry, when I was growing the brand. I probably made hundreds of trips to the area during that time. Then I took on the National Hockey League, and Toronto was solidly on my map. But I'd never thought of golfing there. Canada wasn't exactly known as a golfing mecca. But as Craig described the Oviinbyrd Golf Club in Muskoka, I knew I wanted to go there.

After I got back to the United States, I emailed Craig and said that I wanted to take him up on his offer of a visit to Muskoka to play golf at the Oviinbyrd Golf Club. He was delighted, and I flew north for a visit that would last only thirty-six hours. Craig picked me up at the airport, and we drove deep into a forested area, with a stunning lake dotted with picturesque boats and cottages. It was a scene out of a postcard.

Craig, his wife, Shirley, and I hit it off and had a great time. Later, I calculated that out of the thirty-six-hour visit, we spent five hours golfing and more than triple that time talking and creating the most wonderful friendship. Sure, we played great golf on a course I hadn't even known existed, but the real benefit was the bond. So, if someone invites you into the wilds for a game of golf, always take them up on it.

VOICES IN MY HEAD

Another thing that popped into my head while I was golfing in Tasmania is that, no matter where I'm golfing, I can hear the voices of my golf partners in my head. For example, I'll start to hear Tony, my longtime partner. Tony and I have played in tournaments in Vail and Aspen and Waccabuc since 2006. Often when I'm playing on my own, I'll start to hear Tony's voice. In fact, I always hear Tony's voice. Tony has these phrases that I think are universal where he'll address the ball: "Hello, ball." Or he'll say as he's putting, "Okay, ball, don't be scared of the dark"—which means don't be afraid to fall into the hole.

My friend Steve's voice will pop into my head: "Swing half as hard and enjoy the distance."

And each time I miss a putt, I will hear William: "Missed it by that much." I don't know where these phrases come from, but I love them, and it means my friends are around no matter where I am.

In a long golf game, sometimes your mind can start to drift. That's when I hear the other voices. It's like I have a council of golf buddies living up there, guiding me along. Or it's like a magical database in my brain of past experiences and past shots: *How did I hit the ball? What did my partner say? What did we do next? Did we win or lose the hole?*

A game might take hours, and time has to be filled. On other occasions, I'm in a tight spot and have to pull together memories of what to do. These memories form a magical database in my brain of past experiences and past shots. *How did I hit the putt? How did we win the hole? How did we lose the hole?* These are intense associations that can bring me back through the years to think about a single shot. I'll be on a course such as Tasmania, and my mind will go to all the partners I've had who would have liked to play there, and what they would have thought of the experience.

If I have a philosophy, it's to live each day as if it's your last. In other words, wring as much out of every day as possible. And once I've had a rare experience like I had in Tasmania, I know I want to keep the relationships, and I want to return again. I find that networking becomes that much easier when you understand that the point of a golf trip is not the competition. It's all the great people you meet along the way. Yes, there's a score. But that's not the most important thing to me. The number one thing that I scored on is all the great people that I meet.

One more story. Joe is another one of my best friends. Joe is in my YPO forum. What makes Joe distinctive is he is extremely competitive, and he likes to bet money. I am not much of a gambler, but that is a key part of the experience, and while I have probably only beat Joe a handful of times, it makes the golf so much fun. Joe is also a prolific karaoke singer. So, when he is winning, he starts singing. In fact, many of my friends call him Singing Joe. He likes to sing sixties and seventies songs. He also sings Bruce Springsteen songs—his first cousin is Max Weinstein from the E Street Band.

About ten years ago, Joe invited me and twenty of his other friends on a trip to play at a new golf course called Les Bordes. What made this trip distinctive was that Les Bordes was on the outskirts of Paris. Who knew they played golf in Paris? Obviously I should have. I couldn't wait. I knew a few of the people on the trip, so I was among friends. The experience blew my mind. We arrived in the early morning. Usually when I play golf, I will drink water or Gatorade. At Les Bordes, it was bottles of white burgundy. I am not much of drinker, but when in Paris—right? By the sixth hole, I was over the jet lag and swinging away, albeit a bit tipsy. What a treat.

These experiences bring me back years and even decades. They're part of that connectivity I've been talking about. Recently, playing an extremely tight and difficult course, with the wind blowing hard, I wasn't thinking about golf at all. I was linking the moment to all the tough courses I've played and the partners who were with me. *Oh, he would have enjoyed this. What would he have said?* I was nostalgic for them, but they were there with me. I thought about Marcela—what would she think of this course? *Oh, she'd be more hardcore than me.*

I started chatting with the caddie and got to know him and his story. It really improved my experience of the play. The point is, I'm never alone on the golf course.

THE QUEEN AND KING OF COUPLES GOLF

Marcela and I have been playing in tournaments together as partners or as a couple for more than fifteen years, and we've won some couple tournaments. Some people call couples tournaments Divorce Opens, because the pressure and the expectations can get to some couples. But when we play together, I'm never more relaxed. I know Marcela doesn't judge me for how I play golf and suddenly my shots seem to get better. I know where she likes to hit her shots from, and my objective is to give the next shot that she likes. She likes to be in front of the green so she can chip up. She doesn't like to be in sand traps. Sometimes I wonder if I should just play my golf the way she likes. I would be so much better.

Marcela is very competitive. She wants to win. There was a stretch in 2022 when Marcela and I won a couple of tournaments in a row. I'm happy to be with her, and she has ice in her veins. She clutch-putts when she needs to.

9

WOMEN BREAK THE MOLD

In 2012, when former Secretary of State Condoleezza Rice became the first woman to be admitted to the Augusta National Golf Club, along with financier Darla Moore, she helped break an eighty-year tradition that was long overdue to be broken. There had been a notion in golf that men could not really relax and enjoy the game if there were women around. But Rice, with her prestige and her utter seriousness about a game she had only started playing seven years earlier, was happy to break the mold and dispatch those old ideas to the dust heap of history.

Women are making tremendous strides in the game of golf. Maybe they're not happening fast enough, but today in the United States, there are about 6.4 million female golfers and climbing. The biggest clue to the future is the statistics involving junior development programs. Today, 38 percent of all golfers under eighteen are girls. We already talked about the pandemic effect. In 2021, 37 percent of new golfers were women. Organizations like the Women in Golf Foundation offer training, support, and networking opportunities that are helping female golfers become more visible and more competitive.

Golf gives me the ability to get lost in something I love doing.

—SHELLI BETTMAN,
Golf Advocate

Whether as amateurs or as professionals, women golfers today stand on the backs of some truly great pioneers. Legendary women golfers—such as Babe Zaharias, who broke through during the fifties and sixties; Kathy Whitworth, whose remarkable winning streak (eighty-eight times on the LPGA tour) spanned more than thirty years from the sixties into the nineties; and Annika Sorenstam, often applauded as the greatest female player of all time—inspired generations of young women to take up the sport and helped open doors to women playing.

TOP 5 WOMEN'S WORLD GOLF RANKINGS

1. Nelly Korda, United States
2. Lilia Vu, United States
3. Céline Boutier, France
4. Yin Ruoning, China
5. Hannah Green, Australia

SHELLI BETTMAN—
Golf Advocate, Taking No Prisoners

The most memorable shot I have ever seen came from Shelli Bettman on the Bandon Dunes Golf Course in Oregon. Shelli and her husband, National Hockey League Commissioner Gary Bettman, had invited Marcela and me to take the place of another couple that had to cancel. What an amazing invite. Marcela and I had known Gary and Shelli personally and professionally for more than ten years. Shelli and I got along very well and every time we were together, we spoke about two subjects—politics and golf. Marcela had just started golfing at the time. Gary had been golfing for a number of years and was shooting in the 90s. Shelli was a competitive golfer with a great swing, lots of power, and tons of confidence.

We played all four courses at Bandon Dunes (today there are seven courses). The match was Shelli versus Mike, with Marcela and Gary playing for fun. Let me just say this—I didn't win one match against Shelli.

On our last match, I had a chance to win. We were on the eighteenth hole on Bandon Trails. In my mind, we were tied. Shelli hit her tee shot into a bunker. It was an uphill, 150-plus-yard shot to the green. Most people would hit a short shot to get out of the bunker, which had a high lip. Shelli said she was going to hit her 3-wood—a very aggressive shot. I thought to myself, *Sure, anything you want*, believing it was to my advantage. It was a very-low-percentage shot. Shelli hit the ball, and it went straight to the green. Truly amazing.

She just smiled and said, "I do that all the time." Best loss of my life. A shot I will remember forever.

Whenever I see Shelli, it's my first comment. "How did you make that shot?" She just smiles.

Shelli is a passionate golfer, and she takes no prisoners. She won't tolerate the denigrating attitude toward women golfers that sometimes seeps in at clubs. She's pretty blunt about it. "The fact is, women are completely second-class citizens," she told me. "I have yet to go to a club where that's not true."

Shelli related this story to make her point: "I was at a club—I won't say where. It was probably a par 4, and my second shot was way uphill. I was in a sand trap, about 125 yards off the green. The caddie walked over and handed me a sand wedge. I looked at him. 'You're kidding, right?' He said, 'No, you need to just get out.' I was peeved. 'I don't want to just get out,' I told him. 'I want to get on the damn green.' He replied, 'Well, you can't get on the green.'"

It was the caddie's certainty that bothered Shelli—his contempt for her game. It was the notion that she couldn't possibly know or execute any actions other than just getting out. She wanted to prove him wrong, and she hit it well—it was just off the green. But she never wanted to play with that caddie again.

"I'm very competitive," Shelli told me. "I always have been—and it's not that I'm so competitive against people. I'm competitive with myself. Golf gives me the ability to get lost in something I love doing." As such she deserves to be treated with respect.

It is very important for Shelli to play the game as she wants to play it. "When I started playing, I happened to learn on a course that had no caddies, and it was a blessing in disguise because it forced me to figure everything out about my game—what kind of clubs to use, what kind of shots to hit. It forced me to read the green. I didn't have someone buzzing in my ear. It was liberating.

"Now I have caddies who are used to me. They don't look twice when I grab a 3-wood to get out of the rough. In the beginning, if I took out the 3-wood, they'd say, 'You really should take a 7-iron.' I didn't want to do that and give up yardage." Shelli has become an advocate among the women she knows to find their own comfort zones, and not necessarily listen to a caddie. "I go out with them, and they see me hit a 3-wood out of the rough. I tell them, 'Give it a try. You can do it too.' There are a lot of women who are strong enough to get out there with other clubs and smack that puppy! And when they do it, they're just amazed that they can do it.

"I say, 'What do you have to lose?' I'm very friendly with an LPGA pro at my club. When we went out to play, I got into a trap, and I was near the front lip. I took out my 4-hybrid, and the pro looked at me and asked, 'Really?' I said, 'Yep.' I walked up to the ball. I tilted my shoulders. I adjusted my stance, and I hit the ball. The pro still talks about that shot."

DEBBIE DONIGER—
Championing Women and Never Thinking Twice

I had an opportunity to speak with Debbie Doniger, a professional golfer and master instructor, who started to play golf seriously at the age of twelve. For the past twenty-one years, Debbie has been the director of instruction at GlenArbor Golf Club in Bedford, New York.

Debbie grew up in Greenwich, Connecticut, but her golfing life started in California when her maternal grandparents bought a place in Palm Springs. It was on the grounds of the Tamarisk Golf Club, the site of the Bob Hope Desert Classic (now the American Express). Every vacation, Debbie couldn't wait to visit.

"It was the most fun part of growing up," she said. "I could drive the golf cart, and I could spend time with my grandfather. That's where I was introduced to golf, and the love of golf. I met my first teacher Shirley Spork there—one of the founders of the LPGA." And then Debbie began honing her playing and afterward her teaching career with Jim McLean.

When Debbie was twelve, she announced that she wanted to play on the LPGA Tour. Her plan baffled her friends back home. "Growing up in the northeast in the eighties and loving golf, you were kind of viewed as a total loser and an outcast. Nobody played golf—let alone a girl." So, she had to battle her way into the game. She stuck with it, and she played at the University of North Carolina, Chapel Hill. She was captain of the team from sophomore to senior year, leading them into the top ten. When she was a senior, they won the Atlantic Coast Conference Championship. Today, Debbie is proudly in the ACC Hall of Fame.

"It changed my life. From the very beginning, in every way," she said. "I have friends from junior golf that I'm still very close to. I would never have gone to North Carolina if it weren't for golf. I would never have met the best friends of my life there or been part of the incredible team with the incredible coach."

Her mother begged her to go to business school or get a master's degree. I said: "I don't know what you're talking about. I'm going to make the tour. And I'm going to make a living on the tour."

She also understands that golf turns off many girls and women because it takes itself so seriously. Tournament golf is one thing, but a fun day on the course with friends is just as valuable. She blames the scoring system and the overfocus on par for getting in the way of how people enjoy golf. "If you take away the par goal altogether for social golfers, you'll see a big improvement in their experience of golf. Instead of par, create other goals: How many fairways did you hit? How many greens did you hit? And so on. Those measures become your score."

Today Debbie is an evangelist for the game and all that it brings to the table. "I tell kids there are so many opportunities within golf. You don't have to play the LPGA tour. You can go into media or apparel or research and development, or events. There is a huge array of opportunities."

YOUNG FEMALE CATALYSTS

Across the board, young women from different backgrounds are finding ways to engage in golf for business and pleasure. They are the new catalysts for the sport.

Margaret Wentz and Cailyn Henderson are twenty-four-year-old women's golf catalysts who have been close friends since they played together on their high school golf team. Cailyn is a professional golfer and social media content creator, and together they started a women's golf-oriented apparel business, Fore the Girls. Their idea came from what they viewed as a gap in the market—few options in golf clothing for women and girls, and the options that do exist are unattractive and bland. Their first product hit the spot. The FTG Blossom Bucket Hat is stylish and bright, in six colors. It's a real standout on the course.

In the process of marketing their products, Margaret and Cailyn are attempting to contribute to a change in attitude around women and golf and encouraging girls to get into the game.

HAESHIN LEE—
A Bright Spirit on the Course

Haeshin Lee was born in Seoul, Korea, but she didn't become a serious golfer until she was an adult with two kids, living in New Jersey. Her husband, James, was in medical school and then a busy medical practice, and she had two small children at home. After they joined the local Alpine Country Club, golf became Haeshin's opening to a wider world, her way of getting to know people in a new country. Haeshin and James became friends with Marcela and me, and it's been quite a journey.

"My first time in the US was a shock," she told me. "I cried every day, with limited English and with no family and friends here. I didn't work and James was so busy starting his career. But thanks to James joining a private golf club and encouraging me to take up the sport, I found myself feeling much better with both a new challenge and a new perspective on life. The vocabulary of golf was easier for me to learn. Golf saved my life and my marriage. Through golf, I was able to meet interesting people and gain friends from all different cultures, backgrounds, and business fields."

Haeshin had studied music—she had a BS in music theory at Seoul National University. And she was delighted to find many similarities between music and golf in terms of practice, training, and mentoring. It was also the performance mentality—the desire to get it right. These were all familiar to her from her music experience. Music helped her a lot when she was learning to play golf.

"Was it the rhythm, or was it the precision required?" Both, but the technical comes first. When you're playing the piano and you hit a key wrong, people know. The same is true with a golf swing.

Haeshin met a lot of people through golf, and because she was dealing with language and cultural barriers, it was a constant learning experience for her. She found that in a four-hour game, she could find out the most important qualities of her companions. "Golf is like life," she told me. "In four hours together, you can see their true colors, whether they are selfish, gracious, or caring. You can see a lot of their personality on the course and how they deal with life in general. Golf is a game of integrity, and honestly, that is how I live my life—when dealing with my marriage, raising my kids, and building friendships. I guess that's the reason I play golf and love the game."

Haeshin knows what she's talking about. Everyone wants to play with her. She's a beautiful spirit on the course, and she's racked up golf championships at many clubs, including multiple times at the Alpine Country Club.

Hearing from Haeshin always brings a big smile to me and Marcela. She has that effect on people. We love our time together, and she's good at keeping in touch with people. She embodies that bright, happy spirit I so love to see when I'm out on the golf course. That love of golf, and love of the friends we make through golf.

WHAT A PAIR! (WOMEN POWER)

My favorite photo of all time, which is on display in my golf room, is the photo of Marcela winning the three-day, member-member tournament at Eagle Springs Golf Club in Edwards, Colorado.

At the time Marcela and I had just become members of the club, and we didn't know many people. So, to meet the other members, we let the head golf professional pair us up with others who were looking to meet people. In this tournament, we played five nine-hole matches against other two-person teams. There was a men's division and a women's division.

I had been paired up with a member, so I was all set. Marcela was waiting. And it came down to the day before the tournament when she was paired with Heather from Orange County, California.

Marcela and Heather literally met on the golf course before their first match. They didn't even get to play a practice round together. And as the saying goes, the rest is history.

Heather and Marcela were a perfect match. Two outgoing, charming, strong, competitive women who were in it to win it. From their first match, you would have thought they had been playing together for ten years. They instantly had chemistry and were on top of the leaderboard in their flight. They bonded over life, their careers, their golf, and any other subject. The power of golf bonding was in full effect.

I was doing pretty well with my partner too. We had won our flight, and we had made it to the shootout.

There was a men's shootout and a women's shootout. Unfortunately, my partner and I were eliminated after the first hole in our shootout. Then Heather's husband, Allan, came over and said Marcela and Heather had made it to the final group and were playing the last hole for the championship. Quickly, we raced over in a golf cart to watch them. Marcela and Heather were playing alternate shots, which means that each player hit every other shot until they holed the putt. Heather crushed the drive, Marcela hit the second shot right down the middle, and then Heather hit another shot straight, keeping the ball in front of them.

The other team was doing amazingly well too. They were tied until they made it close to the green. In golf, the shorter the shot, the more your heart rate goes up and nerves can take over. You always hear about professional golfers saying that they can clear their mind. I wish I could do that.

The other team chipped their ball, and it went over the green. Marcela and Heather kept the ball in front of them and only had to get the ball in the hole in two putts and they would win. And they did.

From not knowing each other before the tournament, now they were champions. Heather and Marcela became longtime golf partners, ski partners in the winter, and friends for life. All our children got married, grandchildren came along, and the two of them won the championship again a few years later. Hard to win once, quite an accomplishment to repeat. The most impressive female golf pairing I've ever witnessed.

The truth is that Marcela enjoys playing with me and the family, but she really loves tournaments. "My personality is perfect for tournaments," she told me, and it's true. She can be extremely focused in a way I'll never achieve. "I love strategy," she explained. "If you're losing, you strategize differently than if you're winning. Either way it's fun. So is the challenge. I always ask myself, 'What can I do today?' I love controlling the mental aspects of the game."

However, like me, Marcela enjoys the social side of the game as well. "You can tell a lot about someone's personality when you're playing with them on the golf course," she said. "Even when you've just met. Are they desperate to win? Are they polite? Are they so competitive they try to bring you down? I tend to play with the people I like." This is why Marcela and Heather make such great partners.

When I see the game of golf through Marcela's eyes, I realize the extent to which women are thriving on the golf course. Marcela doesn't experience a woman's place as an uphill battle or something she has to fight for. She simply goes with the flow and enjoys golf for what it is, for the pure enjoyment of being out in nature with family and friends, challenging herself in small ways and large, and engaging in a fun activity with the people she loves.

10

THE LANGUAGE OF GOLF

The language of golf can be spoken with your eyes. The language of golf can be spoken with your hands. The language of golf can be spoken with your reactions. But golf is also awash with terminology. Golf has a unique language that you must learn, no matter what type of golfer you are. The good news is that it is a universal language and no matter where you are playing around the world it is pretty much the same. When you use these terms in speaking golf, you will be in good shape. Here's the rundown on golfspeak from start to finish.

WELCOME TO THE CLUB

When you arrive at a golf course, there are a number of buildings you should become familiar with.

clubhouse   The central building at a golf course that serves as the social hub for golfers, offering amenities like dining, locker rooms, and a pro shop.

bag drop	A designated area where golfers can leave their golf bags upon arrival. The staff will then transport them to the starting area or prepare them for play.
locker rooms	Facilities within the clubhouse where golfers can change clothes, store personal items, and freshen up before or after their round of golf.
halfway house	A rest stop located near the middle of the golf course, offering refreshments and snacks to golfers midway through their round.
beverage cart	A mobile service that delivers drinks and light snacks to golfers on the course, providing convenience and hydration during play.
driving range	An area at a golf course or a dedicated venue where golfers can hit golf balls into an open field to practice or warm up before play.
pro shop	A retail store within a golf course or clubhouse that sells golf equipment, apparel, and accessories, and often offers services like checking in for a round, club fitting, and lessons from a golf professional.

When you go onto a golf course, most of the terms I'm talking about initially will be about the outdoor game of golf. What we're going to find is that the indoor game shares several of the terms in a virtual setting, whereas the outdoor golf courses are in a live setting. Some of the terms that are not always known are actually key. The first one is when you get to a golf course, you need to know where the bag drop is. That's important because you have a very large bag of golf clubs, and you have to drop them somewhere near where you're going to play golf. And then you're going to have to park the car. So, the first thing you typically want to do is find the bag drop. Next, you'll want to know where the clubhouse is, since the clubhouse is essential to all facets of golf. It houses the locker rooms where you can change into your golf clothes, and where you are going to sign into the golf course typically in the pro shop and talk to the person who's going to set up your tee time. If you're going to have any refreshments or food, that's also where the dining room is.

The most confusing part of a new golf experience is knowing where everything is located. I can't tell you how many times I've experienced that—wandering around looking for things. I got lost so often that I started building twenty or thirty extra minutes into the schedule.

THE PEOPLE YOU'LL MEET

There are a few people you will see when you start a round of golf:

starter	An employee of the golf course responsible for managing the flow of play by ensuring that golfers start their rounds at their designated tee times.
marshal	A course official who patrols the golf course to help maintain the pace of play and enforce rules and etiquette.

They will ask you . . .

tee time	A pre-scheduled time when a group of golfers is set to begin their round of golf.
front nine **back nine**	The first nine holes (1–9) and the last nine holes (10–18) of an eighteen-hole golf course, respectively.

And how many people are in your group:

single	A lone golfer playing by him- or herself. Singles often have to navigate the course differently, especially during busy times, as golf courses typically prefer to group players together to maximize the use of the course and maintain a steady pace of play.
twosome	This refers to two people playing a round of golf together. It's a common configuration for friends playing a casual round or when the course is not too crowded, allowing for faster play.
threesome	A group of three players. Threesomes are often formed when a twosome is paired with a single player by the golf course to optimize tee times and course usage.
foursome	The most traditional group size in golf, consisting of four players. Foursomes can be competitive or casual and are a standard configuration for many golf tournaments, leagues, and casual rounds. It's often considered the ideal group size for maintaining a good pace of play while allowing for social interaction among players.

Another thing that is a lot harder than it should be is figuring out who the starter is, and then who the on-course marshals are going to be. The role of the starter is to coordinate the start of play and make sure players get to the tee on time with the group they're playing with.

The tee time is the starting time. Tee times are typically scheduled in increments of four to six minutes. Most tee times are recorded electronically using different apps.

handicap	A numerical measure of a golfer's potential ability, calculated based on previous scores and used to level the playing field in competitions.
stroke play	A format where the player with the lowest total number of strokes for the entire course wins.
match play	A format where players or teams compete on a hole-by-hole basis, with the overall winner having won the most holes.
ready golf	To improve the pace of play, especially in casual rounds, players are often encouraged to play in the order they are ready, rather than strictly adhering to the honors rule. This approach is recommended by many golf associations, including USGA.

What is your handicap? What are the handicaps of those with whom you're playing? And what format will you be playing? Often, you play match play (more on that later in this chapter) while keeping track of how many strokes each player has taken for purposes of maintaining a valid handicap. These days people are starting to keep score through an online system, so your score for each hole goes straight into the app and is recorded. It used to be that you'd play a round of golf and walk to the computer and enter your score. Whether it was high or low, entering a number was a point of pride. It gave you a handicap and therefore legitimacy.

The handicap system is critically important, because the handicap allows golfers to play with one another. A very good golfer with a low handicap—say 5—and a high handicap golfer—say 17—can play together because the low handicap golfer will give the high handicap golfer twelve extra strokes to make the game equitable.

There's a constant banter going on between golfers about whether people are putting in their scores—the correct scores. It's an open question: Do your scores reflect your play?

If you record a higher score than you actually played, you're called a sandbagger, meaning you're sandbagging your handicap and making it artificially high so you get more strokes. On the other side of sandbaggers are people who have vanity handicaps. A vanity handicapper is someone who should have a higher number—say, 17 or 18—but records a 12.

I've often wondered why people would want a vanity handicap that didn't match their play. They'd never be able to win a match or even come close. Their golf partners might feel frustrated. It seems like a lousy plan.

Golf actually has a pretty good system for finding these people out because scores are recorded and put into an app called GHIN—the Golf Handicap & Information Network. All golfers worldwide have a variation of GHIN—one of the reasons I could easily play golf in Uruguay.

The reason that the handicap system was initially used was because there was a lot more betting in golf. In the early years, golf betting was synonymous with what is called "the nineteenth hole," which is drinking. (There are eighteen holes on a typical golf course. Golfers affectionately call the bar in the clubhouse the nineteenth hole.) But the handicap has become intrinsic to enjoying golf. Often, the first question you're asked is, "What's your handicap?"

As a golfer who has had a handicap higher than fifteen for my whole career, I've always had a higher handicap. And yet, on any given hole,

I could get a par or birdie, and people would say, "You're not a real 15." I'd wonder to myself if they knew what a 15 handicap looks like. A real 15 has some holes and some battles. As you become a better and more consistent player, your handicap drops lower.

Where the handicap becomes important is when I have a 15 handicap and I'm playing a 5 handicap on ten holes, I'm going to be given a stroke or a one-shot advantage. If it takes me five strokes to finish the hole, it'll be a five net four—counted as a four. Sometimes to speed things up, we call that fifty-four (54).

The only issue that I really have with handicapping is the word, which is derived from horse racing. Is it the right word? In today's world, *handicap* has a negative connotation. You can't escape that. For someone like me, with a high handicap, it reinforces the point, almost putting me in a negative light. I don't think handicaps should be judgmental, and yet the whole concept of handicapping is judgmental. Even when I look up the definition of *handicap* in the dictionary, it reads: "a circumstance that makes progress or success difficult."

Is that really what golf means? I think we need to come up with a more positive word for *handicap* that reflects the reality that it is an index that allows everyone to play together.

THE FORMAT MATTERS

How many people are in your group? Are you a single? Are there two of you? Three? Four? Typically, golf is set up to go in fours, at least in the United States. In New Zealand they're more likely to go in fives. But if you play golf in fours, an average eighteen-hole golf round will take four and a half hours. After that you need to decide what type of match—stroke play or match play. You're always going to record each stroke you're playing, how many strokes it takes you to complete each hole. But you also might want to have something called *match play*. There you play on a hole-by-hole basis, with the winner winning the most holes.

Many of my most memorable tournaments have been match play tournaments. If you win the hole, you get a point, if you tie, you each get half a point, and if you lose, you get zero. At the end of nine holes, the scores are calculated and whoever wins the match gets an extra point. You get the extra point because you won! And often that extra point can make all the difference if you are in a competitive flight.

In most of the tournaments that I play, there are usually thirty to forty golfers. To make things more competitive, they are divided into flights (a term for golf team) with five or six golfers per flight. These flights are like divisions in football. The main difference in these tournaments is that the flights are ranked by ability (handicap), so that golfers of similar ability are playing against one another. Therefore, in any given tournament of forty golfers broken into eight flights, there can be eight flight winners. Those flight winners will play in some sort of playoff to determine who is the overall winner of the tournament.

I am usually a good partner for a golf tournament, because I have a relatively high handicap and, from time to time, can make a par or birdie on a hole. That has allowed me to win several tournaments. The statistician in me might say that if you play enough tournaments, you are bound to win one. But I don't think that's how golf works.

Tony and I often won our flights at Waccabuc Country Club and Maroon Creek Club in Aspen because, on those magical weekends, we were playing well. Golf has an unusual term called "ham and egging." That's when two people are playing together as partners and only one of them is playing good golf. The other one is playing poorly. Most of the time, Tony was playing the good golf, and every so often when he was off on a hole, I would play well. That was frustrating to our opponents, but it was very good for our scorecard.

One of the most legendary teams I ever saw play was the team of my friends William and Sam. In almost half the tournaments they played at the Waccabuc Country Club, they won their flight. In fact, they won so often and so consistently, the golf committee came up with a rule that if you won your flight the previous year, they would reduce your handicap—and William and Sam still won. How did they do it?

William and Sam had been childhood friends—they could complete each other's sentences. They had an ease of playing with each other that was palpable. Waccabuc is William's home course, and he played extremely well there and knew all the greens. Sam had a relatively consistent game of golf, but mostly he had an ability to get in the heads of his opponents. This was way before the "back off" challenge on TikTok, when golfers would insult one another to see if they could get their opponents to back off. It is more like stand-up comedy than anything, but golf does require some concentration. When I'd play against Sam, sometimes I would bring a set of ear plugs.

My most memorable loss was when my friend Joe and I were playing in a tournament at his home club, Quaker Ridge, in Scarsdale, New York. It was our second year; the first year we had won our flight. I am not sure it was "ham and egging." It may have been just Joe. We'd come in second place in the whole tournament after a long shootout—and we were playing to win. We were one point behind the team above us. They had to make two putts that were in the back of the hole, which means they were downhill putts. And if the putts did not go into the hole, we'd win.

Our opponents were old-timers, kind of salty, in their late sixties or early seventies. They had won their fair share of tournaments over the years. You could tell they'd been together for a long time. They were emotionally confident although they weren't especially low handicappers. But we were playing a match game, so it didn't matter how many strokes were made for each hole; it just had to be fewer than our opponents.

On the fifteenth hole, which was the toughest hole on the course, one of our opponents made an impressive shot to the back of the green. It was an extreme downhill putt, and the only question was whether it would go directly into the hole or way past it. The putt was that fast. And he made it.

They beat us by one stroke and went on to win the flight. They did not go on to win the whole tournament. But after playing golf for two straight days, our entire tournament came down to this one putt. I can recall many times playing with my regular partners when these putts matter a lot, and that's when the ice has to start running in your veins.

If I have a weakness as a golfer, and I think all my partners would tell you, I don't always have the ice running in my veins. I get nervous and sometimes I can't block it out. And so my friend Joe, when the pressure is on, asks to make my putt, even when it's the friendliest game, because I will often miss it. And he sinks his every time. Joe is best under pressure.

This is what makes golf so exciting. You can practice your drive and you can practice your short game and even your sand game. It all comes down to whether you can make the putt at the critical time.

IT'S TEE TIME

Once the round begins, you will go to the first tee box and agree on the tees you will be playing, which will be designated by tee markers:

tee box	The starting point of each hole where golfers make their first stroke.
tee markers	The different sets of tee markers on tee boxes are used to accommodate players of various levels, offering them the right distance from which to play the hole. These tees are typically color-coded, although the specific colors and their associated distances can vary somewhat from course to course. Here is an example from one of the courses that I play at frequently.

- BLACK TEE: These are often the farthest from the green and are intended for highly skilled golfers.
- BLUE TEE: Usually set for experienced amateur golfers with a low to mid-handicap.
- WHITE TEE: The standard tees for the average golfer, offering a moderate level of difficulty.
- GREEN TEE: These are the forward-most tees.

Some courses may introduce additional colors, like silver or red, to further customize the playing experience for different groups of golfers.

Determining who will tee off first is done by giving the honors. The concept of "honors" when teeing off is an important tradition and part of golf etiquette, determining the order in which players begin their play on each hole. Here's a detailed look at how honors work in different contexts:

having the honors	Earning the right to be the first player to tee off on a hole.
how the honors is determined	At the start: On the first tee, the order of play can be decided by random choice, by the players' handicaps (lowest goes first), by a flip of a tee or coin, or through mutual agreement. Subsequent holes: After the first hole, the player who had the best score on the previous hole earns the honors and tees off first. The next best score tees off second, and so on. In the event of a tie, the order from the previous tee is maintained among those who tied.

etiquette and respect	Honors is a part of the etiquette of golf, showing respect for the performance of fellow players. It's a recognition of a player's achievement on the previous hole.

The initial shot you hit off the first tee will be your drive. If all goes to plan, the second shot will be your approach, then maybe a pitch, approach lob, or chip if you don't land on the green, and then putt the ball into the hole.

If you think that your shot may be heading in the direction that it could hurt someone, yell *"Fore!"* When I first started playing golf, I thought, *"For what?"* Later I realized that it was *fore* as in something that is in front of.

drive	A long-distance shot typically taken from the tee box.
approach	A shot intended to place the ball on the green.
chip	A short-range shot played from near the green, intended to loft the ball into the air slightly before it lands and rolls toward the hole.
pitch	A shot that is longer than a chip, designed to fly higher and land softly on the green.
lob	A very high, short shot intended to clear an obstacle and land softly.
bunker shot (or sand shot)	A shot made from a bunker, usually using a special club called a sand wedge.

| mulligan | Informally, a "do-over" shot allowed by fellow players after a particularly poor shot, not counted in official play. |
| fore | A warning shout used to alert other players or spectators that a wayward golf ball might be heading their way. It's a courtesy to prevent injury. |

From each shot you hit, your ball will land in a number of different places. Each one has a name. And within that place, it has a quality of position called a "lie."

fairway	The area between the tee box and the green, typically well-maintained grass that makes it easier to hit farther shots.
lie	The position of the golf ball when it comes to rest; also refers to the quality of that position (e.g., good lie, bad lie).
green	The area surrounding the hole, with very finely cut grass, where players putt.
primary rough	The first cut of rough. It's longer than the fairway but shorter than the secondary rough.
secondary rough	Thicker and longer than the primary rough, making recovery shots more difficult.
heavy rough	Very thick and unkempt grass areas, sometimes found farther from the fairway. It's the most challenging type of rough, often significantly impacting play.

bunker (or sand trap)	Hollowed-out areas filled with sand, usually near the green or fairway, that pose an additional challenge.
water hazards	Bodies of water like lakes, rivers, or ponds that can catch errant shots.
out of bounds	Areas marked as beyond the play area of the golf course. Hitting the ball out of bounds incurs a penalty.

Shapes of Shots

waggle	A series of small movements or adjustments made by a golfer before taking a shot. It's part of the pre-shot routine that helps the golfer relax and prepare for the swing.
slice	A shot that curves dramatically from left to right (for a right-handed player), often unintentional. It's typically caused by an open clubface and/or an outside-in swing path.
fade	A controlled shot that moves slightly from left to right (for a right-handed player). Unlike a slice, a fade is usually intentional and offers more control and predictability.
draw	A shot that curves slightly from right to left (for a right-handed player). It's generally seen as a desirable shot shape for its ability to gain extra distance.

| hook | A shot that curves sharply from right to left (for a right-handed player), often more severe and less controlled than a draw. |

What's in Your Bag?

The standard advice is that you need fourteen clubs, but that hard and fast rule is changing. I spoke with Greg Pattison, owner with his wife, Monica, of Gott Golf, a custom golf club fitter and builder in Denver, Colorado. Pattison got into the business through his love of golf. "I was always one that enjoyed working on golf clubs and figuring out how to make them better for me and my friends," he told me. "It was a passion that turned into a major career, helping others enjoy the game as much as I do."

For Pattison, it's all about individual needs, especially for beginners. "One of my favorite things to tell people that come and see us is that money doesn't dictate that you play this game any better," he said. "You can enter the game and get the equipment that's right for you at a minimal cost." That's a big deal, because expense is often cited as a barrier to entry, and Pattison insists that doesn't have to be the case. "Depending on your goals, you can obviously take it as far as you want, but it doesn't have to be an expensive barrier of entry."

He starts by challenging some rigid assumptions. "The rules of the game allow up to fourteen clubs in your bag, but there's no reason you have to start with that many. It's about starting with the right clubs that help you learn and progress in the game. So, it could be eight clubs. I think a beginner shouldn't have more than eight clubs in the bag. As you start to play the game and get comfortable, you'll start looking at what's club number 9? What's club number 10? And so on. When I taught my wife this game twenty-plus years ago, we didn't have all the technology now available to us in the many different types of clubs. So, my wife learned the game with a driver, a 5-wood, a 7-iron, a pitching wedge, and a putter."

driver	A long club for distance.
putter	For an easy roll toward the hole.
wedge	A club that gives you loft if you need to hit over tall grass or to get over a sand trap.
woods	For distance on the fairway: 3-wood = 125 to 240 yards 4-wood = 110 to 220 yards 5-wood = 105 to 215 yards 7-wood = 90 to 170 yards [According to Dick's Sporting Goods]
irons	Power and distance: 2-iron = 105 to 210 yards 3-iron = 100 to 205 yards 4-iron = 90 to 190 yards 5-iron = 80 to 175 yards 6-iron = 70 to 165 yards 7-iron = 65 to 155 yards 8-iron = 60 to 145 yards 9-iron = 55 to 135 yards [According to Dick's Sporting Goods]
hybrids	A combination club that provides both distance and accuracy.

The question of clubs brings up the issue of affordability, which is a constant theme in new player development. I spoke with Kenyatta Ramsey, vice president of player development for the PGA Tour, and he emphasized his commitment to eliminating barriers for new players and the coaches who support them. His special focus is on encouraging player development from historically black colleges. "It comes down to resources, you know. God bless them, man! I didn't realize how much work that these college coaches do. Sometimes they are doing four and five different jobs, including being a part-time parent to the students. They have to raise money for equipment and technology."

Kenyatta is a big fan of the "pass it forward" programs, especially for people donating used clubs so students can afford to play. Speaking to him got me thinking about how many people have old clubs in their garages. It's time to pass them on so these kids can play. (That's my public service announcement.)

SPECIAL RULES

As you are approaching the green, you may encounter different areas of the course where specific rules apply, often leading to penalty strokes if a player's ball enters these areas. These stakes are color coded to distinguish the type of area they mark and the rules that apply. Here are the primary penalty stakes you'll encounter:

red stakes (lateral hazard markers)	Red stakes or lines indicate a lateral water hazard. If a ball lands in an area marked by red stakes, the player has several options for proceeding with a one-stroke penalty. These options include playing the ball as it lies (without penalty); dropping a ball behind the hazard, keeping the point where the ball last crossed the margin of the hazard directly between the hole and the spot on which the ball is dropped; dropping within two club-lengths of where the ball last crossed the edge of the hazard, no closer to the hole; or replaying the shot from the original position.

yellow stakes (water hazard markers)	Yellow stakes or lines designate a regular water hazard. The relief options for a ball in a yellow-staked hazard include playing the ball as it lies, dropping behind the hazard with the point of entry between the hole and the drop point (with a one-stroke penalty), or replaying the shot from the original position (also with a one-stroke penalty).
white stakes (out of bounds)	White stakes or lines indicate out-of-bounds areas. A ball hit out of bounds requires the player to take a stroke and distance penalty, meaning they incur a one-stroke penalty and must play another ball from as close as possible at the spot from which the original ball was last played (essentially hitting again from the same position).

Understanding the meaning of these stakes and the penalties associated with them is crucial for golfers to make informed decisions on the course and to adhere to the rules of golf. Note that specific local rules and exceptions might apply depending on the golf course, so when in doubt, it's a good idea to consult the course's rule sheet or a course official.

When You Reach the Green

putt	A shot made on the green where the ball is struck gently enough to roll into the hole.
lag putt	A long putt aimed more at getting the ball close to the hole rather than trying to make it in one shot. It's a strategic putt to ensure an easier next shot, ideally leaving the ball within a "gimme" distance.

| gimme | An informally agreed-upon short putt that the other players allow to be considered holed without being played. It's typically granted when the ball is very close to the hole, and it's almost certain the player would make the putt. |
| grain of the green | Refers to the direction in which the grass on the green grows. The grain can affect the roll of the ball, especially on putts, making it slower when putting against the grain and faster when putting with the grain. |

Types of Golf Scores on Each Hole

par	The number of strokes a skilled golfer is expected to make to complete a hole.
birdie	One stroke under par.
eagle	Two strokes under par.
albatross (or Double Eagle)	Three strokes under par.
bogey	One stroke over par.
double bogey	Two strokes over par.
triple bogey	Three strokes over par.

The scoring system can be a bit suspect. There are two ways golf is scored. One is how many strokes it takes to get from the tee box to sinking the ball in the hole. If you hit a drive and you hit a 6-iron and approach shot, and then you hit two putts that take and you get on the green, and that takes you two putts to get in, that's a four. Unless it's not. It depends on the arbitrary decision of what is par, and what numbers are below and above par.

I have often wondered whether par is part of the problem with golf. I understand that par is a comparative metric. I know how par is determined. I know how a combination of holes can add up to par 72 or par 71. My issue is not with the literal number that is par. My issue is with the concept of par.

Par gets into my head. And on each hole, the first thing I think about is the par. Is it a par 3 or is it a par 4? Some holes can even be a par 5.

Par is completely judgmental, based on how many strokes somebody thought the hole should take. Did it take you four and then you got to par? Or did it take you five and you got a bogey, or took you six and you got a double bogey, or you got three, so you got a birdie.

In tournaments, they assign each hole a number, and they add up all the strokes you take over the course of four days. If you have five less than the next guy, you beat them by five strokes.

The whole par, bogey, double bogey, birdie nomenclature, while maybe nominally helpful, can mess with your psyche as a golfer. Even the great Tiger Woods used to have something called a Tiger Par. Tiger's father, Earl, would say to Tiger, in effect: "But for you, if you get there in five, that's a par." And so they use the system in a totally different way. And sometimes I think that the enemy of golf is this system because golfers feel they have to get the hole in a certain number of strokes or they've failed. That's why they use match play in so many tournaments. The match is between you and your opponent, one against the other. You only have to be one stroke better to beat your opponent on a hole, and one hole better to beat your opponent at the game.

Instead of par, create other goals: How many fairways did you hit? How many greens did you hit? And so on. Those measures become your score.

—DEBBIE DONIGER,
Professional Golfer and Master Instructor

PERFORMANCE METRICS

Because I count everything, as you get deeper into golf, there may be some metrics that you want to keep. Both "Greens in Regulation" and "Fairways in Regulation" are crucial metrics for evaluating a golfer's performance, highlighting the player's accuracy and consistency throughout a round. Achieving high rates in these statistics is often a good indicator of a golfer's potential to score well.

Until you get there, at least you will know what people are talking about.

greens in regulation (GIR)	This is a statistic that measures how often a golfer reaches the green in the recommended number of strokes (two strokes less than par), resulting in an opportunity to putt for birdie or better. It is a key performance indicator in golf, as it demonstrates a player's accuracy and skill in both driving and approach shots. A high GIR percentage is often correlated with lower scoring.

fairways in regulation
Similar to GIR, this term refers to the percentage of tee shots on par 4 and par 5 holes that land in the fairway. It's a measure of a golfer's accuracy off the tee. Hitting fairways in regulation is critical for setting up the opportunity to hit the green in regulation, as playing from the fairway usually offers a better chance to control the ball than playing from the rough or other challenging lies.

Types of Golf Courses

parkland course
A golf course characterized by lush, manicured landscapes, plenty of trees, and often inland settings. These courses resemble traditional parkland and may include water hazards and strategic bunkering.

desert course
Designed to fit into arid environments, these courses feature natural desert landscapes, limited turf areas, and are often found in places like the southwestern United States. They require specific strategies due to the unique terrain.

links course
Originally referring to courses on the sandy coastline of Scotland, these courses are defined by their coastal location, undulating fairways, deep bunkers, and a lack of trees. The term *links* comes from the Old English word *hlinc*, meaning "rising ground or ridge."

| executive course | A shorter golf course designed for quicker play, typically featuring more par 3 and par 4 holes than standard courses. It's ideal for beginners, those looking for a quick round, or experienced players wanting to practice their short game |

The Golf Formats

There are many different formats that can be used when you play golf. When you are playing in a tournament, typically the organizer will group teams into groups of two or four players.

Team Formats

scramble	All team members hit from the best previous shot.
shamble	Like a scramble, but after the best drive is chosen, players finish the hole with their own ball.
best ball	Each player plays their own ball; the lowest score counts as the team score on each hole.
alternate shot	Teams of two alternate hitting the same ball.
pinehurst	Both team members tee off, then switch balls for the second shot, choose the best ball, and play alternate shot from there.
four-ball	Similar to best ball but played in teams of two in match play format.
foursomes	Two-player teams hit alternate shots with one ball.

| Scotch foursomes | A mix of alternate shots with each player teeing off and then deciding which ball to play. |

Individual Formats

stroke play	The total number of strokes taken over the course determines the winner.
match play	Players compete hole by hole, and the player with the most holes won is the winner.
stableford	Points are awarded for each hole based on comparison to par.
modified stableford	Adjusted point values encourage aggressive play

Less Formal Games

In less formal situations, these are the games that we play in casual games.

Nassau	Three separate matches in one round (front nine, back nine, and overall).
skins game	Each hole is worth a set amount, with the best score winning the hole; ties roll over.
six-six-six	A round divided into three different match formats.
wolf	A rotating three-versus-one game where the "wolf" can choose a partner or go it alone after teeing off.

Bets

While playing a round of golf, there are many different types of side bets that can be made through all phases.

trash or junk	Players earn points for various mishaps.
hog	A player can declare themselves the "hog" to double their win or loss on a hole.
snake	Involves putting, where missing a short putt adds a penalty until another player misses.
baseball golf	Scoring similar to baseball, where certain outcomes equate to singles, doubles, etc.

Trash of Golf

ferret	Earning a point for holing out from off the green, not limited to chipping, can include bunker shots.
whales	Making a birdie or better on holes with water hazards.
crownies	Making par or better after hitting the ball out of bounds or into a provisional situation.
sandy birdies	A "sandy" that results in a birdie or better, adding an extra layer of achievement.
acey-deucey	Making a net 2 on any hole, which can include actual aces (holes in one) or net eagles on par 4s.
Hogies (or Hogan)	Winning a bet by hitting the green in regulation but then two-putting for par, a blend of prowess and slight disappointment. Named after Ben Hogan.
lumberjack	Making par or better on a hole after hitting two or more trees.
rockies	Making par or better after hitting a rock or rocky terrain.

NOT ABOUT GOLF

cactus	Specifically for desert courses, making par or better after coming into contact with a cactus.
rainbows	Making par or better on a hole where your drive had a significant arc or "rainbow" trajectory.
dew sweeper	For early morning rounds, making birdie on the first hole.
ghosties	Making par or better on a hole without hitting the fairway or green in regulation.
conquistadors	Conquering the hardest hole on the course according to its handicap rating with a par or better.
Sherlock	Finding and playing a ball that was initially deemed lost but was then found within the search time limit.
blind squirrels	Finding something good unexpectedly, like making a long putt you didn't think you'd make.
Skywalkers	Making par or better after hitting a shot that unintentionally goes extremely high.
thread the needle	Hitting a successful shot through a narrow gap between obstacles like trees.
circus putts	Making a putt that curves dramatically or takes an unusual path to the hole.
dances with wolves	Making par or better on a hole with wildlife visibly present.
escape artist	Making par or better after declaring an unplayable lie anywhere on the course.

tin cup	Going for it on a risky shot over a hazard instead of playing it safe, and succeeding in making par or better.
phoenix	Making par or better on a hole immediately following a double bogey or worse.
dragons	Making a net birdie or better on the most difficult hole of the course, as declared before the round.
giraffes	Making par or better on a hole where your tee shot had an unusually long hang time.
bounce back	Scoring par or better on a hole immediately following a bogey or worse.
Atlas	Carrying the team on a hole in a best ball or scramble format, where your score is the only one that counts for the team.
leap frogs	Making par or better on a hole by skipping the ball over water.
vultures	Making a birdie or better on a hole immediately after someone else in your group scores a bogey or worse, "feeding" off their misfortune.
pirates	Successfully stealing a hole in match play that your opponent seemed certain to win.

These playful challenges can be tailored to the specific rules or situations of a round, adding an extra layer of fun and camaraderie to the game. They encourage players to focus on various aspects of play, from precision and recovery to simply enjoying the quirks of the game.

THE JOKES OF GOLF

There is a joke in golf called the "Golfer's Dilemma" that will always make a room of golfers laugh no matter how many times they've heard it. It isn't a bellyache laugh though. It's a nervous laugh because it rings true for many people. They know someone who they suspected had done it, the thought had gone through their mind. This is the joke, which I'm crediting to Gary Mule Deer:

You are playing for the club championship. You and your opponent are tied after seventeen holes. You have the honors on the eighteenth tee and proceed to hit a drive dead center 250 yards down the fairway. Your opponent hits it right into the woods. After trying to help him find his ball for ten minutes, he tells you to go ahead and hit your second shot. He will look for a couple more minutes and, if he can't find it, he'll go back and re-tee. You hit a beautiful second shot ten feet from the cup. Just as your ball hits the green, you hear, "Found it!" and your opponent's shot comes screaming out of the woods and lands only inches from the cup. As your opponent approaches the green, you now face a dilemma. Do you pull the cheating bastard's ball out of your pocket and confront him, or keep your mouth shut?

When you spend four hours on the golf course, you have to find ways to fill dead time. Making jokes is one of those time-honored ways. I learned this lesson from my business, and it applies to golf.

During the pandemic, my office on West 33rd Street in New York City was closed. I went from a space with twenty people on Tuesday, March 10, 2020, to one that was basically empty on Thursday, March 12. I remember the last meeting that I did from my office was a Zoom meeting with a client who had some staff outside of Washington, DC, and some staff in Santa Monica, California. The meeting started at 5:00 p.m. New York City was emptying out, the streets were silent. But the call went on because I think the people on the West Coast weren't yet 100 percent up to speed on what was happening in New York City.

After that meeting ended, I knew that working would never be the same. I had three issues: (1) The team I had was young. It was the first job for many of them. How would they adjust to working from home? How could I put into place a structure so they would know when to work? (2) Many of my team didn't know "how" to work. The office was much more than just a location. It was the place where we collaborated, we discussed things, where we used a mentoring system to teach them "how" to work. To be part of a team, to contribute, and to foster professional development. (3) My team didn't really know the new way to communicate over Zoom. While video conferencing had been around in various forms for the previous few years, it was new. There was no training for how to communicate on Zoom. We turned on the camera and the room appeared. The meetings with the presentations were exactly the same as if we were there. But this felt different. We wouldn't just use Zoom occasionally. We were going to use Zoom all the time.

Something had to change. I knew we had to train people to communicate on Zoom. But how? They were gone. And then I remembered. Over the years, I had a friend in LA named Desiree Gruber. When you meet Desiree, you never forget her. She lives in the future at the intersection of "What's Next?" and "Let's Make It Happen." One day near the end of one of our calls, she said that she had to leave early because she was taking up stand-up comedy lessons with her son. I never forgot that because I thought it was so cool.

That's what was needed for my team. The challenge of Zoom was that everyone on my team was alone, in a room, staring into a computer screen, with a light in their faces. Unlike being one of many where they could disappear into a crowd in a conference room, they were all out there in Zoom.

Zoom meetings had long pauses, awkward moments, people staring at one another. Particularly at the beginning of the pandemic, no one knew what to do. It was horrible. Seconds seemed like minutes, minutes like hours. It was so bad.

And that's when we hired Desiree's stand-up comedian coach, Jo Scott. Jo Scott was an amazing stand-up comedian, improvisation expert, and wonderful person. Once a week, for sixty to ninety minutes, Jo taught us how to be stand-ups. How to break the ice, make chitchat, have a few jokes. And suddenly our Zoom calls became more relaxed. We started to look forward to them. They weren't a grind. We'd develop new material and take three to five minutes before the meetings to try out our material as people gathered. It completely changed the dynamic.

The golf course is the same way. There is a lot of time in between shots. You spend more time talking and getting into position to play golf than you spend playing golf. A repertoire of chitchat, jokes, current events, and business topics is absolutely required, or you will not make it through. The more you have some topics ready to go, the quicker the awkward moments dissipate.

THE TRUTH ABOUT A HOLE IN ONE

I want to talk about the mythology of the hole in one. Even if you've never played golf a day in your life, you've heard of a hole in one and you know what it is. A hole in one is one of those rare terms that has transcended this sport, I think there are a few terms that do this—such as *kickoff* in football, *home run* in baseball, or *slam dunk* in basketball.

Maybe you didn't know that the odds of making a hole in one at any given time are extremely steep. According to the National Hole-in-One Registry, the odds of the average golfer making a hole in one are 12,500 to 1. Broken down even further, here are the odds of:

- Tour player making an ace: 3,000 to 1
- Low handicapper making an ace: 5,000 to 1
- Two players from the same foursome acing the same hole: 17 million to 1

- One player making two holes in one in the same round:
  67 million to 1

Each year there are 450 million rounds of golf played in the United States, which is approximately 25,000 to 30,000 per course. Each course reports between ten to fifteen aces per year. Basically, that means a hole in one is scored once in every 3,500 rounds.

Bottom line: Holes in one don't happen often. Only 2 percent of golfers score an ace each year, and the average number of years those lucky ones play before they score is twenty-four years. That's a worrisome statistic for me, because I started playing golf in my early twenties and I'm now fifty-five, so I'm due for a hole in one. The good news is that golfers between fifty and fifty-nine account for 25 percent of the holes in one. I'm in the right age group. I have four more years to make it. On the other hand, these stats are meaningless because hardly anyone, including people in their fifties, make holes in one. But I'll keep hoping, and maybe include my wife in the picture. Sixteen percent of holes in one are made by women, and the average age is fifty-five. So, Marcela and I are both due to make our holes in one!

There's always hope for people like me. The average handicap of a golfer who makes a hole in one is fourteen.

THE DRESS CODE OF GOLF

The last thing to discuss is the dress code in golf. As you can see from some of the interviews in this book, the golf dress code is going through a transition. The reason is simple. Golf is no longer the sole domain of the old-school, country club set. It has reached popular culture. And popular culture has a lot of ideas about proper style.

There's no reason you need to wear a collared shirt when you play golf, and yet, that's the dress code when you play. In most places, you have to wear golf shorts, or you have to wear slacks. You can't play golf in workout clothes or wear blue jeans. And I sweat. There's a certain level of style that we're going to have that's appropriate to the environment. Yet in some circles a more individualized and casual style is attracting a new generation to the game, and that's a good thing. We're seeing a transformation as more people of color, younger people, and more women play the sport. Gradually there's a transition in the way that people dress. It's something we're already observing in the larger society—casual Fridays and fewer suits and ties. Certainly, the pandemic contributed to this shift.

People want to relax, be more comfortable, and express themselves more. One of my clients is Crocs, and their motto is "Come as you are." Crocs are an extreme comfort, but also full of self-expression, with so many different varieties. If you want to wear your Crocs with socks, you're more than welcome.

The typical dress code for a golf course aims to maintain a tradition of decorum and respect for the game. While specific requirements can vary by golf course and country, common elements of a golf course dress code include:

1. Collared shirts: Men are typically required to wear collared polo shirts. Women may wear collared shirts or golf-appropriate fashion tops.

2. Slacks or golf shorts: Golfers are usually encouraged to wear slacks or golf-specific shorts. The shorts should be of an appropriate length, typically near knee-length.

3. Golf shoes: Footwear should be golf shoes with soft spikes or flat-soled sneakers designed for golf. Metal spikes are often prohibited to protect the greens.

4. No denim: Jeans and denim material are generally not allowed on the golf course or in the clubhouse.

5.   Hats and visors: While hats and visors are commonly worn to protect from the sun, they should be golf-appropriate and worn with the brim facing forward.

6.   Skirts and skorts: Women may wear skirts or skorts that are designed for golf and of an appropriate length.

7.   No athletic or workout clothes: Clothes that are too casual, such as gym shorts, tank tops, and T-shirts, are usually not permitted.

Some courses, especially private or more upscale venues, may have stricter dress codes, requiring items like a jacket and tie in the clubhouse. On the other hand, public or municipal courses might have more relaxed guidelines. It's always a good idea to check in advance the specific dress code of the course you plan to visit.

I say this with a huge caveat: Stay tuned! There is a revolution coming in golf attire, and it's already visible in informal settings.

10 THINGS I HATE ABOUT GOLF

1.   Why do they call it a handicap? I don't feel handicapped when I play golf.

2.   Par. I feel like I am judged on every hole even before I start.

3.   The shame of nine holes. I hate that if I play only nine holes, I have to make an excuse for why I didn't play eighteen. In all situations, nine should be fine.

4.   Players who cheat. Honor counts.

5. Players who take the game too seriously—play slow, grind over every putt, talk it out.

6. Players who take too long putting. There needs to be a putting clock like a shot clock or play clock.

7. Playing in bad weather. Why do people insist on playing golf when it is cold? Or windy? Or rainy?

8. Players who have a no chitchat policy.

9. Bad snacks on the course. Golf is a healthy sport with unhealthy traditions.

10. The old, complicated rules. Golf is a simple game with complicated rules.

11

THE GAMES OF GOLF

My favorite room in the house is my golf room. I'd never wanted a typical "man cave," where I could drink or smoke or do whatever people do in man caves. I wanted a room dedicated to golf that I could enjoy with my family and friends. I set up a simulator, just like the one I'd admired on HBO's *Entourage*. That series came out years after I had built mine. It could be snowing outside, but I'm golfing inside. And, of course, there's the big TV so we can watch sports.

Home golf rooms with simulators are a relatively new phenomenon, but they're getting hot fast. The golf room has become one of the features people love building into new homes—a place to congregate, watch sports, and play golf.

Sometimes on a long conference call, I'll set up the speakerphone (old days, it was a button on the phone attached to the wall; today it is just my iPhone strategically angled on a cabinet) and do the calls while I was hitting balls. It's a way to multitask, especially on calls where my presence is needed but not so much my input. No one hears the thump, thump, thump in the background.

The simulator can be deeply satisfying. Trust me. On a winter day, playing on the simulator, you get that same euphoric dopamine rush you feel out on the course. Here's another secret I've discovered: I'm a 20 handicap on the golf course, but I'm a 10 handicap on the simulator—which gives me hope for my outdoor game. Here's the rub: On the simulator, you never lose a ball. Every lie is perfect. Every shot goes somewhere—you're just hitting into the wall. So, it's not a true test. That doesn't mean it isn't fun!

During COVID, the golf room was the most popular room in the house, always being used by my twenty-five-year-old son who was living with us, my wife, or me. It was the most used room in our house other than the kitchen.

To walk into the golf room is like walking into Mike's photo museum of golf. There are photos everywhere of all my golf friends, all the faces, all the trips, all the tournaments. I even frame the scorecards from tournaments that I or Marcela have won.

GOLF AT THE INTERSECTION
OF HOSPITALITY AND ENTERTAINMENT

An Addictive Environment

I knew that the future of golf was in simulator golf. It had all the elements of golf that were great—the dopamine rush that came from hitting the ball in the air combined with all the modern technology that was only getting better every year.

One Saturday evening, I joined friends to play at Topgolf in Holtsville on Long Island. Holtsville is a demographically diverse community with very solid family values. It's a big deal to go to Topgolf on Saturday nights—every one of 130 bays is filled. I saw some guys arrive with their serious bags. They were there for a heavy workout. At the same time, the bay next to us was a birthday party for a nine-year-old girl. They were playing an Angry Birds golf game and having the time of their lives. And I realized I was seeing the future of golf right before my eyes.

Topgolf, owned by Callaway, is the latest popular iteration of golf—a sports entertainment complex that offers a high-tech golf experience for all ages and skill levels. There's food and drink and music and a hitting experience tailored to whatever your needs and desires might be.

I sat down to talk with Topgolf CEO Artie Starrs. By the time he joined the company in 2021, Artie had been in the mass branding business for most of his career, recently as Pizza Hut Global CEO within Yum! Brands. He knows a lot about popular trends. In addition, he admits to being a golf fanatic. "In all areas, golf changed my life," he told me. His experience somewhat echoed mine and included his whole family. "I met my wife through golf, I made the best friends in the world through golf. I got into a better college through golf. Now I have my dream job because of golf."

His take on the importance of Topgolf is simple: "We're taking an aspirational game and bringing to the forefront the best thing about it in the easiest and most accessible way. Think about it. If you ask golf enthusiasts why they love golf, most of them won't even tell you it's the game of golf they love. They'll say it's the quality time with their friends and families."

All of this is wrapped into an experience that is exciting and even addictive. Artie told me that most people play for about two hours. "It's pretty fun. The thrill of hitting a good golf shot is a highlight. They get hooked." He argues that it's much more exhilarating than a traditional golf range. "It's multistory. We have lights. We're playing loud music. The food is good. The technology and the gaming are clearly addictive."

In the world of golf, Topgolf represents a major new direction and expanded access. "There are two ways to sell golf," Artie said. "The first way, you say you need about four and a half hours. You've got to have a warm-up period. You've got to read the rule book. You've got to carry around fourteen clubs. You've got to wear a collared shirt. Boom, boom, boom, boom, boom. The second way is an invitation to show up, try it out. Hit some balls, have a burger and a beer. Play a video game while you're doing it. Without a doubt, the second way creates more new golfers.

A HOT URBAN VENUE

Five Iron cofounders Jared Solomon and Mike Doyle first met in the back of a custom suit store in New York City where Mike gave private golf lessons on a simulator. It was perfect timing for Jared. After law school he'd gone to work on Wall Street, and he was finding the social scene boring—the "same old dinners at Smith & Wollensky" and the like. He wanted something more interesting to do.

Jared had never played golf growing up, but he loved the data and golf play at Mike's back-of-the-store simulator lessons. Mike had a decent lesson business there, which organically turned into an after-work social event. Everyone had a great time, socializing and hitting balls on the simulator. As time went on, Jared and Mike measured the success and began to think about what they could do with a bigger place, including a kitchen and bar, leagues and coaches, in a wildly entertaining atmosphere. Their concept was to marry golf with entertainment and the free-flowing abandonment they saw in New York street art. It would reject the old ways in large part, because they didn't know about them. They didn't come out of that culture. "We didn't know that you're supposed to use maroons and dark greens, and look like a country club, with music at a low volume. We were interested in making a place that we wanted to go to."

And so, Five Iron was born in 2017. They added Jared's wife, Katherine, as chief legal officer and took on a fourth partner, Nora Dunnan, as chief operating officer. And they set out to capture the emerging zeitgeist. "There's a perception that golf is hard, and I think when you're outdoors on a driving range, it really is," Jared said. "But there's sort of a magic to a simulator where you're in this safe space that demystifies the game. It also changes what success looks like. From a pure entertainment standpoint, what success looks like is things blowing up on the screen, and bells and whistles going off. It changes the way that people think about golf and makes it accessible."

That accessibility creates a positive adrenaline rush for players. "Everyone can get the ball in the air in ten minutes," Jared said. "We create that feeling of euphoria early in the experience and that leads to people being addicted for life."

From the outset, they made the decision that they would not have a club or membership-only system, although there would be a membership option, which created a loyal customer base. There would be no dress code, no stuffiness. Five Iron would be a welcoming place for everybody, whether it be golfers, nongolfers, or the golf curious. The opposite of the exclusivity that was part of the history of golf. "Most people view it like the top of a funnel—how do you get somebody at their first shot?" Jared said. "But the truth is, what we do is not just the top. It's also taking those at the middle of the funnel and turning them into real golf fans. We take the person who maybe played with their dad a little when they were a kid, or a couple times with their buddies in college, and all of a sudden you're taking lessons at Five Iron. Then you're joining a club. You're becoming a consumer of the sport. We've heard thousands of those stories. They try it here, and then they get obsessed with it. That's how the sport grows."

By 2024, Five Iron had grown to twenty-four locations, including a new flagship at Grand Central Terminal. That's when Shake Shack founder and restaurant innovator Danny Meyer placed a big bet on the company, investing $20 million. He saw in their vision the same thing that had always motivated him—the drive to make a great experience more accessible.

Meyer also could relate to the Five Iron customer. Golf had never been his game, and by the time he decided to learn, he found the prospect somewhat daunting. He was a very busy guy and had scant time to play, much less travel to a course on the outskirts of the city. He started taking lessons with a golf pro at an indoor simulator and found the experience fit his needs perfectly. He could see the future of golf right in the urban heart of Manhattan.

BOONE SCHWEITZER—
Trashing the Old Ways

If you want real comfort on the course, why not trash the old rules—or turn them charmingly upside down? Boone Schweitzer, a prominent realtor and sportsman in Snowmass Village, Colorado, vividly recalled the origin of Trashmasters, his over-the-top concept that has introduced a wildly counterintuitive element to the game, while raising massive funds for scholarships.

It was during the mid to late eighties. Boone played a lot of golf with his buddies at the Snowmass Club, and they were getting bored with the traditional games. One day, they started to joke around. "Somebody hit a tree, and I said, 'I think you're working on a barkie,'" Boone remembered. "Then somebody hit a ball into the water, and we said, 'Let's call that a drinky.' And from this very humble beginning, we started our first tournament in 1992. I scared up twenty-four local guys to play. The idea was that we would reward the strange and bizarre events. It just took off and we started adding trash events. Today we have about twenty-six."

The casual concept grew into a nonprofit organization hosting tournaments to raise money for scholarships. Boone chaired the Trashmasters Tournament for twenty-five years, and he's still involved. He's proudest of the fact that more than a hundred kids have graduated from college with the Trashmasters scholarships. But he's also proud of having imagined a way to play golf that is pure fun—not the hard slog that golf often is for people.

"Notice the demeanor of the guy on the first tee," he told me. "It's upbeat, positive, jovial. And then it deteriorates during the day. Coming off the eighteenth hole, that's a different guy. With Trashmasters, most people take off their competitive hats and put on their fun hats, taking the game lightly, and laughing at each other. It's a strange combination. It's very competitive, but the players are laughing the whole time."

From the outset it is hilariously different. It starts with the oath you have to take. Boone explains, "When I show up in the robe and wig and have everybody raise their right hands and swear to play trash, the whole trash, and nothing but the trash, and we blow off the cannon, it kind of sets the tone."

Boone acknowledges that a Trashmasters Tournament is a boisterous event, kind of an inverted Masters. Boone admits that he came up with the name Trashmasters when he was watching the Masters. It got him into a little bit of trouble.

As he described it to me, one day he went to his post office box in Snowmass Village. There was a large envelope, and the return address was a law firm in Washington, DC. Inside was a legal complaint from the Masters against the trademarking of Trashmasters.

Boone had a remote office at the time, and he took a walk into the village to clear his head. He came across a friend, Doug Pruessing, one of the founders of Trashmasters. Doug saw his gloomy face, and asked what was wrong. Boone showed him the letter.

"Let me have this," Doug said. "I'll take care of it."

Doug, who had deep pockets, enlisted a top trademark law firm in Washington, DC, to go up against the Masters in a lawsuit. Boone was named in the suit.

"We were in court with the Masters for several years, and we got a lot of press," Boone said. "We got a lot of bank. We finally settled out of court, and we got to keep the name and register the trademark. It was all good. I can talk about this now, because Doug passed away a couple years ago. He was one of my mentors—a top guy and a great player. Doug viewed this as a classic David and Goliath story."

Boone boasts: "I can take a 16 handicapper—we have high handicappers all the time. We have four flights. We've got women. We've got senior championship, but a 16 handicapper can be holding that trophy and putting on a yellow jacket and feeling good about it."

For me, golf is a way to meet people, socialize, have a few good laughs, and get a beer at the end of the day. That's it. I don't play to be competitive. I'd rather have fun.

—BOONE SCHWEITZER,
Founder, Trashmasters Tournament

A few years ago, Trashmasters came up with a "Boonie," where the player can double the trash points. "I've seen guys do it," Boone laughed. "It's like they won the British Open!"

The bottom line for Boone? His philosophy of the game is simple: "For me, golf is a way to meet people, socialize, have a few good laughs, and get a beer at the end of the day. That's it. I don't play to be competitive. I'd rather have fun. All in the spirit of the game we call golf."

ON THE RADAR

"The question we asked ourselves was, if the Doppler radar can track a missile or projectile, maybe it can track something as peaceful as a golf ball."

That's Klaus Eldrup-Jørgensen speaking. Klaus is CEO of Trackman, a twenty-year-old Danish startup that invented a device that uses Doppler radar to track the trajectory of a golf ball from the moment it connects with the club to when it comes to rest. It then provides real-time data to golfers either on a laptop or smartphone, to help improve their game while on the course.

I'm a technology nerd. I love anything that puts a new spin on things, and the Trackman innovation signals a mini revolution on the golf course. It's the pure intersection of entertainment and science. When you see that little orange box on the course, you know that science is happening. As Trackman presents it, "We are limited only by the laws of physics in our search for answers to the question that has guided us since day one: How can we make it more fun, more engaging, and more efficient to practice, play, and improve."

Like many of these stories, this one is completely unexpected. Before changing his career and cofounding Trackman at the age of forty-five, Klaus was a medical doctor and a director in the pharmaceutical industry. Nothing related to golf. But he'd always loved golf.

"I played golf since I was a kid and won the Danish championship for juniors a couple of times," he told me. "I played the Eisenhower Trophy as an amateur, played on the Danes National team, and so on. So, [I] played golf from about ages thirteen to twenty-five. But then I had to focus on my education as a medical doctor, and that was the end of serious golf."

Klaus's brother was very involved with a friend's business, which included four big driving ranges in Europe—two in London, one in Glasgow, and one in Stockholm. They were probably the largest ranges in Europe at that point, all doing very well. Both brothers had a small investment in the company, and together with their friends they had an idea for how to increase participation at the ranges. What if you could track a golf ball in flight and retrieve data about it? The result would be more fun and a more efficient practice session. It was a simple idea, but it struck at the heart of a need. "We'd see people hitting golf balls all day, and we wanted to add something more to the experience," Klaus explained. "And then we looked around, and we could see that in the military industry they used Doppler radar to track missiles and projectiles." One of the leading companies in the world for Doppler radar, a company called Weibel, was located forty-five minutes from where they lived.

In 2003, they pitched the owner of Weibel, saying, "You have a technology, and we have an idea." Over several meetings, they talked about doing a joint venture, but the owner never really believed in the idea. He wasn't a golfer, and he didn't see the advantages. "He was not super keen," Klaus said. But at every meeting he had sitting next to him Fredrik Tuxen, who had been head of research and development for fifteen years. Fredrik was enormously skilled, doing radars for military applications for NATO and the US military and the like. Weibel was selling these radars all over the world. He was also a golfer who understood golf and its needs.

After several months of getting nowhere, one evening on an impulse Klaus called Fredrik. "I know we haven't spoken before outside of meetings with your owner," he said, "but we're getting nowhere. It looks like this isn't going to happen with your company, and I wondered if you wanted to join us. It would mean basically starting from scratch."

Fredrik was interested enough to talk, and Klaus asked him three critical questions: The first was whether he had a competitive clause that would prevent him from working with them. The answer was no. The second was whether there were any patents they needed to be aware of? The answer was no. And finally, was it possible to develop a smaller product? At that point, the systems were huge, weighing hundreds of kilos and costing millions of dollars. Could they bring down the technology to the level of golf? Fredrik believed they could.

"Fredrik was brave," Klaus said. "Within forty-eight hours he returned and said, 'I'm on board,' which is pretty amazing when you consider we didn't really know each other. But he decided right then to quit his company and join us. And it's been a fantastic relationship ever since."

Once they developed the product, the excitement came from traveling around and demonstrating it. The best way to sell the product was to go straight to the range. "I still recall some of the places. Fredrik was setting up the radar. I was hitting a 6-iron, and the only thing they could do was have somebody run around in the field, looking for the pitch, identifying the pitch, and then measuring it. Then imagine the difference. We set up the unit behind the player. I hit a golf shot, and it was immediately tracked and recorded exactly. We could measure the ball. But we could also tell them the launch angle, the descent angle, the apex point—everything they wanted to know to be more efficient. So, that's how it started. That's how we built the business in the first few years."

That building process operated like a pyramid. At the top were the equipment manufacturers. Once they embraced the technology and used it as a measurement tool to develop new clubs, it achieved a level of credibility. The second level was the players. When the best players in the world use your technology, people will trust you across the board. Next were the tournaments. The little orange box became a familiar sight on the course. Finally, the clubs and the people—and finally the simulator world, which introduced Trackman to the masses.

When simulator golf entered the picture, it was the marriage between fun and science. Trackman is a perfect fit. Klaus is convinced that indoor golf is the way to grow the game. For one thing, it makes the game easy and fun. "It's not that easy for a newcomer on the golf course," he observed—something I already knew. "You know, people dress in a certain way. They speak their own language. They know how to behave, with all the secret codes. It can be pretty intimidating if you're not one of them. So many people fail to take up the game because of the intimidation factor. Then you take indoor golf. You have a beer, there's music playing, people around you are laughing. You can dress any way you like. There is no barrier to entry. So many more people are getting into the game this way. Trackman fits right in. It was actually our original idea, going back twenty years: Go to a golf range, hit golf balls, get data, improve your game, have fun. Look at your statistics, be addicted, come back."

JEFF SMITH—
Embracing Old School and New School

Earlier I mentioned Jeff Smith, the director of instruction at the Vintage Club in Indian Wells, California, and the Director of Instruction at Pine Canyon in Flagstaff, Arizona. He has devoted more than 30,000 lesson hours in his twenty-six-year career as a PGA professional and is widely known for his successful teaching methods for many different skill levels of players.

Jeff has a reason why golf simulators have taken off: It's a new form of golf. "It takes the emotion out of golf, because the entire thing is contrived," he said. "You don't have any uphills. You don't have any downhills. You don't have any balls above your feet. You don't have any balls below your feet. You don't have any thick rough. You can always get a clean shot. There are no impediments to your club touching your ball. You're also in a static environment. There is no wind in your face, and there are virtually no distractions, except for your buddies and the clink of ice in glasses."

Jeff and I have spoken in the past about the best hope for growing golf. It's a conversation that shows the rift between old school purism and new school adventurism. We agree on one thing: Golf is a cultural force. But the nature of the culture depends on whether you're old school or new school, because those two schools are looking at the game differently.

"There are people out there who don't want any music on the golf course," Jeff said. "They're disturbed if someone two holes away is playing music on a speaker. But those guys two holes over want something different out of the game.

"I think the Topgolfs of the world—the indoor golf venues—are also changing the face of golf. They're bringing people to the game in a different way, sometimes competitively with leagues. In many ways, indoor golf and golf simulation are changing the way people approach golf and what they get out of the experience."

> There's sort of a magic to a simulator
> where you're in this safe space
> that demystifies the game.

—JARED SOLOMON,
CEO, Five Iron

And sometimes, these alternative venues are popularized out of necessity. Jeff gave an example. "I had some clients from Japan. In Japan space is limited, so golf is rarely played on an expansive golf course like we have here. It's played at a range or a practice facility. Golfers hone their skills, and that's the whole game for them. They're very serious about it. They want to get good at the strike, the flight, and the distance. That's their enjoyment. They've actually created pleasure in this form of golf, because it's rare to have the money or clout or time to actually go to one of the few golf courses available. When they come to the United States, they can't wait to get on the golf course, and they play all the time."

Jeff has a pure love of the game that manages to embrace both schools, which is kind of the way I feel about it. "I enjoy golf for its silence and solitude," he said. "I enjoy golf for its challenge to me personally, and I enjoy it when I'm with a group and they're playing music. I have fun with it either way because I'm trying to satisfy every side of myself with the game of golf."

That means being open. "I can't say to myself, 'I don't want to be with a serious golfer because I just want to have fun.' Or vice versa. There are many versions. Some bring in the solitude and the focus, and some bring in the social fun. It's important in my job to make sure that everyone gets to enjoy the game the way they want to enjoy it."

PART 3

BUSINESS
AND PLEASURE

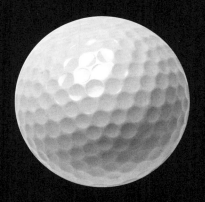

12

"DO YOU GOLF?"

Some of my favorite golf friendships started as business relationships. The projects ended, but the golf endured for years. I don't necessarily seek out golfers. But I've found that when you do business with someone and you build trust, you find out what hobbies they have, what they're interested in, and people learn the most about somebody. Of course, you see their character, you see how they keep their composure, how they interact with people. Golf is an extension of that.

On the golf course, once you run out of idle conversation, you begin to learn what's on people's minds, what keeps them up at night. A deeper bond begins to form. Because of my business as a problem solver, I get into some unusual conversations. I remember golfing with a guy who owned a hundred hair salons. I didn't know anything about hair salons, but he asked me a lot of branding and marketing questions, and that was familiar territory. If there's nothing else, conversations default to politics—something I've known a lot about over the years. When I was working for political figures, people would always want to talk politics.

I spoke with Jimmy Spencer, a sports entertainment executive at The SpringHill Company, LeBron James's entertainment development and production company. Jimmy said that many business conversations start with the question, "Do you golf?" It's a connector, a point of bonding. It can also be a point of pride. "If you play regularly, you have a bit of an edge because it's not an easy game," Jimmy said. "The question 'Do you golf?' is the code for 'Are you part of this special group that I'm part of? That does this special thing together?' Just this morning I was on the phone with a friend of mine, Michael Redd, who played in the NBA for the Milwaukee Bucks for some years and on Team USA with Kobe. During those years, his first question was, 'Do you golf? We've got to go golf together.' And I immediately knew that this was an opportunity for us to spend real time together and get to know each other." They became close friends.

Jimmy also noted that the invitation to play golf is meaningful in a unique way. "It's not 'Let's get coffee' or even 'Let's get lunch.' It's 'Let's go hang out for a half a day.' That's a big deal."

Golf allows people to interact in a more cordial, collegial way. It takes down the barriers and helps them be more authentic. There's nothing more authentic than swinging a golf club. You're out there, you can't hide it. You instantly see the result. Did the ball go up? Did it go in the hole? And it doesn't matter much after that. Forget the score. They just want to know how you played. Did you play fast? Were you pleasant to be with? Do you want to engage? Golf changed my whole perspective on the world.

If you play golf with someone, you'll get to know them better than working with them for ten years.

—ARTIE STARRS,
CEO, Topgolf

As I became more involved with golf, I brought more people into the game. It has become this cycle: *I like golf, I find people who like golf, golf finds people who like me, and my network builds.* People always say business gets done on the golf course, and that might be so, but it's not because you go out there planning to do business. It's because there's a lot of time to chat. Swing, walk, drive. There's five minutes. There are going to be about two minutes in between where you have to fill time. And once you've asked somebody how the kids are, you start talking about issues. My golf course talk is fun. We talk about politics, we talk about current events, we talk about what's going on at home. Everything comes out on a golf course.

One of my favorite golfers is a woman named Polly Flinn, a dynamite marketing executive I met very early on in my professional career. I don't know why, but it took us more than a decade to figure out that we both loved golf. Polly is the first one who took me golfing at the Grant Park course in Chicago. Even though I grew up in Chicago, I had never golfed there before Polly took me. That started our golf relationship. Over the decades we've been on wonderful trips with our spouses to the Kohler Resort and Whistling Straights golf course where the PGA Championship and the Ryder Cup have been held. Our professional connection turned into a very satisfying golfing relationship.

My golfing friendship with Polly is one of my most enduring relationships. Polly is a much better golfer than me—she has won numerous club championships—but we play straight up from my tees—meaning without handicap strokes. That evens things out a bit. There is a lot of golf banter during our matches, but there is also reminiscing about our hometown Chicago, and our mutual love of politics. Polly has been one of my best business advisors, and I have worked with her on projects. She was the first friend to visit Marcela and me at our place in Punta del Este. Polly and Marcela enjoy each other's company and the three of us have fun rounds of golf, although they'll sometimes gang up on me. That's okay. I can handle it. Many of my golf friends have played with Polly in New York and Colorado, and it's always a great experience.

Polly likes to take photos, and our matches are well documented. Hands down, my favorite memento is the note she sent me after we played in New York at Liberty National and Bayonne one July, and I beat her in both matches. Polly included a crisp $100 bill. The framed photo with her note and the Benjamin has a place of honor in my golf room. It was my best day!

THE BEST INTRODUCTION

Steve Gilbert is the chairman of Gilbert Global Equity Partners, an avid golfer, and a member of Golf Digest's Rater's Panel. His introduction to golf came during a winter in New Zealand when he was invited on a boat trip with a group that included a famous movie star. At one point, in the Bay of Islands, the star felt bored. "Let's go play golf."

Steve replied, "You know I don't play golf."

"I know, I know," he said, "but I need someone to come with me." So Steve agreed, figuring he could put on some shorts and running shoes and get in a few-mile run while the star played. He was also curious because the star was known to be a great golfer. It was a regular topic of conversation on his television show.

As Steve watched him hit balls, he was amazed to see him spraying them all over the place. Steve knew enough to recognize that this wasn't good golf. "I don't get it," he said. "You're supposed to be a great golfer. You're terrible!"

The star laughed. "It's a lot harder than it looks. You try." He motioned Steve over and said, "Here's a seven iron, and I'm putting down two balls. There's the green. See if you can hit a ball onto the green."

"Okay," Steve agreed, thinking, how hard could it be? "I took the seven iron and hit the first ball. It went right into the ground. The second ball skirted off somewhere else. I looked at my companion, and being a competitive guy, I said, "Two years. Ten thousand dollars. The charity of your choice."

He said, "Done," and Steve embarked on a mission to learn to play golf. He started to play, and he was terrible at first, but he kept at it. He won the bet, too.

In a sense, every game was a good game to him. He could be philosophical about it. He noticed that some golfers liked to complain about their "bad luck." He had a different perspective: "Please give me all my bad luck on the golf course," he said. "Let the ball take that one-in-a-million bounce the wrong way into the water. Just keep the bad luck on the golf course, and away from the doctor's office, the operating room, the courtroom, the highway, and all the other important locations. As long as the bad luck is on the golf course, I'm fine with it."

Most of all, Steve appreciated the wonderful opportunities for camaraderie.

One day he found himself at Seminole Golf Club in Juno Beach, Florida, with a powerful older trio—an iconic businessman, a billionaire investor, and a well-known chief executive and author.

"They all lived in Florida, and it was their regular game. We warmed up. We played golf. We had a nice lunch at Seminole, and I came home, and my wife asked, "How was your day?"

I said, "It was good. We had interesting conversations. We talked a lot about business. Afterward, I was sitting at my computer when it dawned on me. If I'd called any of these men's offices and said, "My name is Steve Gilbert and I'd like to hang out with you for six hours—and by the way, could you bring along your famous buddies—it would have been preposterous. Yet, that's what had just happened."

Today Steve continues to play often. "I'm going out today," he told me when we spoke. I don't even know who I'm playing with today. But it will be three CEOs, and we're going to be talking about supply chain. We're going to be talking about interest rates. We're going to be talking about politics, leadership, philosophy, the law, regulations, AI, and climate change. What's that worth to a person? I think quite a lot."

MUSICAL SERENDIPITY ON THE COURSE

When my friend Jay Hass was getting his start as a young portfolio manager at the private bank of Brown Brothers Harriman & Co., he was also learning to play golf. His boss was a member of Merion Golf Club in Philadelphia, a club with a distinguished history—and a challenging championship-level course that many of the firm's clients were eager to play. As Jay's game improved and he spent more time around the sport, he noticed that more and more of his clients and friends were doing the same. Business conversations often turned to the latest PGA Tour tournament or courses he and his clients had played. It was almost a language of its own, outside of business, that formed quick bonds.

A guitarist and pianist since childhood, Jay had an interest in the music business, and he noticed that many professional recording artists complained about getting ripped off by their business managers and advisors. Since Brown Brothers had a pristine reputation for integrity and professionalism, with very good investment results, he had an idea. Maybe the firm could build a business focused on this niche. He also noticed that many performing artists played golf on their off days while out on tour. Philadelphia was a great music town; maybe he could meet some artists for a game while in the area. Jay's boss was happy to take them to Merion, as long as they would play fast and obey club traditions. (No hotel room trashers, please!)

Through an introduction from a mutual friend, the first musician Jay played with was Yes keyboardist Rick Wakeman, who loved golf. They arranged to play at Merion. Jay was a little nervous about Wakeman's rockstar-long hair. That might be a problem at the club. Jay asked the mutual friend about it, and he shrugged it off. "He plays the fancy clubs all the time. He puts his hair up under a hat. It'll be fine." And it was. They had a delightful day.

Over the following few years, Jay began to meet more musicians for golf and formed lasting happy memories. After hosting Ed Rowland of the band Collective Soul, Jay came into the office a few days later to find a large box. Rowland had sent a gorgeous Yamaha acoustic guitar, signed by all the members of the band, which he cherishes and plays to this day.

One day in 1993 Jay got a call from the author Michael Bamberger. Michael's golf book *To the Linksland: A Golfing Adventure* had been well received. (More about Michael later.) Michael told Jay that an attorney in Athens, Georgia, had written him a very nice letter saying how much he enjoyed the book. The letter writer, Bertis Downs, was an avid golfer. He also happened to be the lawyer for R.E.M. Bertis was coming to Philadelphia in advance of the band's next tour and was looking for a game. "He seems like such a great guy," Michael told Jay. "I'd love to take him golfing." But Michael was going to be out of town. He asked Jay if he'd be able to step in and host. Just from their correspondence, Michael sensed that Bertis and Jay would get along well and that there might be a business angle as well. Jay said, "Sure, I'm in town."

"From the moment we stepped off the first tee, something clicked," Jay said. "We talked about everything. The similarities were striking. His late father was a Presbyterian minister. My late great grandfather was a Presbyterian minister. He had lived in Richmond, Virginia. My mom's from Richmond. So we found all these points of commonality that had nothing to do with business, nothing to do with music. Meanwhile we were enjoying this lovely round of golf. Just the two of us on a beautiful afternoon."

Over thirty years later, Jay and Bertis are in touch almost every week. Jay is poetic about the evolution of their relationship. "The friendship I made that day with this beautiful person, all because he wrote Michael out of the blue, which led to a four-hour conversation between two strangers . . . where else, how else does that happen? It means the world to me."

And it happened because of golf.

A HOT JOB SKILL

A headline in the *Wall Street Journal* in June 2024 caught my eye: "A Killer Golf Swing Is a Hot Job Skill Now." The article by Callum Borchers went on to describe how companies are eager to hire strong players who know how to do business on the golf course. This is one of the outgrowths of the pandemic, which gave rise to remote or hybrid working arrangements. Why not the golf course. As Borchers put it, "People who can smash 300-yard drives and sink birdie putts are sought-after hires in finance, consulting, sales and other industries, recruiters say. In the hybrid work era, the business golf outing is back in a big way."

Business and golf can form a happy partnership. But how do you get there? I spoke to GlenArbor director of golf David Gagnon about how to make golf part of your business journey. It's like anything else. You put in the time to develop better communication skills, or better writing skills, or better sales skills. Gagnon has seen many young business professionals putting in the time to learn to play golf, so they'll have that extra advantage. Maybe if you're lucky, you'll find someone like David who can coach you and give you an edge. Make it a career skill—one of the most valuable assets you can build for your professional and personal life. You don't need to be a great golfer. Just achieve basic competency.

David asked, "If you were thinking about learning a skill, and you knew there was no downside, and only positives would come from it, why wouldn't you do it?"

But it's not just skills in an abstract sense. It's a quality of sociability you need to develop as well. David knew me from almost the start, and he saw me golfing with many business associates over the years, including Mayor Mike Bloomberg. He shocked me recently by saying: "I'll tell you, Mike, if you'd been a jerk on the golf course, you never would have progressed. Your success had nothing to do with your golf game. It had to do with who you are on the golf course."

GOLF FRIENDS IN THE EXTREME

My friend Jay Hass is also a marathon runner. He likes a challenge and he's in great shape. So, I invited him to join me for what is considered the Ironman of golf—the Solstice at Bandon Dunes Golf Resort in Oregon on the Pacific Coast. On the longest day of the year, Bandon hosts a solstice event where players play four eighteen-hole courses in a single day—seventy-two holes and about twenty-six miles, and you have to walk the whole course. No carts.

Jay and I started at 5:30 a.m., in a marine-layer fog on the Bandon Trails golf course. No warm-up swings. Just get up and hit. Putts within eight feet were gimmes. We each had a caddie, and we had times we had to be at the next course. Like a marathon, we were eating our meals while we played. And in the course of one day, we had all types of weather—fog, bright hot sunshine, drenching humidity, twenty-mile-per-hour winds, and a chilling dusk round to end on the Bandon Dunes course. When it was all over, I had broken 90 on each course. I only lost a few balls, and if I ever get the chance to do it again, I will sign up in a second and so will Jay.

THANKS, GREG

I was inspired to do the Solstice by my stepfather, Greg. He had always told me that his dream was to play three rounds of golf on the longest day of the year. He did it once. That got my competitive spirit up. I wondered if I could do all four rounds. I was a bit of an extreme golfer. I'd done thirty-six holes in a day—eighteen in the morning and eighteen in the afternoon. When I was an Ironman, I could play endless rounds of golf. So, playing golf was so much easier than Ironman.

Greg, the man who introduced me to golf and with whom I spent countless enjoyable days on the golf course, passed away in 2021. It was a real blow, but I had only happy memories of our times together. Greg had a store in Chicago called Reuss Sport and Ski, so he came out of a sports-oriented background. Funny thing, I never asked him how he started golfing. But he was so happy to pass it on.

When I started to do my pegboard and launched my adventures in golf, it's like Greg and I switched roles. I got much more into golf and was more intense. I only broke 80 one time in my life. I went golfing with Greg and my brother-in-law at a course near Greg's house, and it just happened—I shot a 77. Because playing with Greg was like coming home. I was always aware that he was at the center of my golf origin story. And I never came close to that score again. When we started playing tournaments, I revered him as my golf guide. And then our roles changed, and I became his. I have a picture of us playing a golf tournament together on display in my golf room.

Greg was the only person who would go hole by hole with me on the phone about any course I played and talk it through. Even if he had never played the course, Greg wanted to know the layout, the club, the distance, and the result. Endlessly.

Looking back, I don't know if he ever really cared. But he always made me think he did. Greg always took my calls and never hung up until I had exhausted myself from talking. He never said he had to go. I just ran out of steam.

The last time I played golf with Greg was at Whistling Straits, the site of the PGA Championship. It was part of the Kohler Resort, and there were six golf courses next to one another off the shores of Lake Michigan in Sheboygan, Wisconsin. I was in Chicago for a wedding, and I planned a thank-you for Greg after all these years. He had introduced me to golf, and I wanted to invite him on a golf trip. So, it was me, Marcela, my friend Polly, and Greg. We were going to play as much golf as possible in one day at Kohler.

Most of the Kohler golf courses are walking only. Wisconsin isn't that flat, and it isn't that cool. Walking thirty-six holes for a day of golf was going to be some good exercise.

I was concerned because Greg was a cancer survivor. But Greg said no problem. He loved to walk. It would give him time in between shots and allow us to catch up. At the time, I was training for my second Ironman Triathlon in Kona, Hawaii, so I was in pretty good shape. Marcela walks seven to ten miles a day, so she is in good shape, and Polly is a former marathon runner, so she had no problem.

We started on Whistling Straits, which is long and hilly. Greg was doing fine, hanging in there. The next course was Great Wolf Run. A little more straightforward. But hard, long, and some hills. I noticed Greg's shots weren't as crisp. He didn't say anything. But I could tell. This was a big day of golf for him. I went to get him a cart. And we were back in business.

That night, we all met for dinner. I hadn't allowed my mother near the golf course (that was sacred ground), but I did let her come to dinner. Of course, that made Greg happy. And Polly wanted to ask her embarrassing questions about me. I tried to stop her from answering, but my mother is my mother. And besides, let's see how I do when my kids' colleagues ask about when they were kids. Will I be able to keep my mouth shut? Probably not.

I just wanted to be with Greg. And do what he and I loved best—golf. And then talk about golf. It was my gift to him, but selfishly I think it was my gift to myself.

I can't really remember if I ever golfed with Greg again. I doubt it. I always thought we had so much time. His cancer was gone. Next, I thought we would go to Pebble Beach and then Augusta. I had so many ideas of places we could golf. Always next year. Next year never came. He died. I never thought it would be so soon.

I am constantly aware that Greg had a huge impact on my family. He got me into golf. I got Marcela into golf. My son is very much into golf. I often wonder, where would we be without golf? I'm fifty-five years old. I don't know what I would've done with my time without golf. Our lives, our plans, our trips, center around golf. All because Greg put that club in my hands one day long ago.

I still have Greg's clubs. No idea what to do with them. Sometimes I think I should frame his driver and put it on my wall. I would call it the Slicer. I don't think Greg ever hit a straight drive. He always lost thirty yards because his drive sliced.

Greg always said hit fairways and greens. Or maybe he said hit them long and straight. I can't remember. He used a lot of golf clichés. It made me smile and love him more. He was so cute in his passion for golf. He could play with professional athletes in pro-ams at the Western Open, and he could play in his Sunday foursome at Old Wayne, which was the municipal course in his neighborhood.

Maybe in the great golf course in the sky, he finally straightened out his drive. I just wish he was back on the tee box with us.

Thanks, Mom, for bringing Greg into our lives. He was a keeper.

13

THE BEST WAY TO DO BUSINESS

In 2001, I started working for a new client in New York, someone who would come to have a lasting impact on the city that will be felt for generations. Mike Bloomberg was already well known in the technology and publishing arenas and was a tremendous philanthropist. He was quickly changing the world and changing technology. And he was planning to run for mayor of New York City, which is where I came in.

When I started doing research, I landed on his appeal: Bloomberg stood for innovation. He stood for doing things differently. That was the sweet spot for targeting voters. I was excited to be working for such an innovator. I knew it would be a great ride. As the world knows, Mike won that election in the wake of 9/11, and he was a very popular mayor.

At the time I was getting pretty serious about golf, still waiting to be accepted at Waccabuc. But a new club, GlenArbor in Bedford Hills, was looking for members, and the application process was different than at Waccabuc. I was able to get in through my references.

I had a very high handicap, and when I went to the meeting with the founders and told them my handicap, they looked a bit scandalized. "Well, that's going to have to get lower," they said.

"Absolutely," I said eagerly. "That's why I'm joining this golf club. I wanted to lower my handicap."

Being on the ground floor at GlenArbor wasn't the usual golf club experience. We were all new members, and the clubhouse hadn't even been built yet. Marcela and I started to golf as an everyday activity. Marcela would pick Matthew up from school, and they would go to GlenArbor and golf. And while there wasn't a clubhouse, there was a mobile home that served as the pro shop, and they always had a plate of cookies. So, Matthew would get cookies. Marcela began to really see herself golfing. We were both taking lessons.

When our kids were young, I had very strict golf rules. I could golf Monday through Friday, all I wanted. No golf on Saturday and Sunday, because that was family time. And I was good with that. Although, looking back, I am shocked that I was. And I started to meet many people at GlenArbor. Eventually, we got into Waccabuc, but we still had a restricted membership for a couple years. So, we were playing a majority of our golf at GlenArbor. And many of my golf friends were also members of GlenArbor. So, we were meeting there to play a lot of golf together.

When Mike Bloomberg ran for mayor, he had to resign from all New York City country clubs where he was a member, and he joined GlenArbor, which was conveniently located for the mayor. So, Mike and I had something else in common—we got to know each other on the golf course. He'd sometimes play with his daughter Emma while I was playing with my family. On occasion Mike and I would play together, and it was wonderful time spent with the mayor.

As always happens, I got to know him a little better on the golf course. I saw him in an environment that was comfortable for him, hitting great shots. I could recognize the precision, thought, and commitment that were characteristic of him in the rest of his life. He was always looking to improve his swing and correct his mistakes, and sometimes we'd end up playing until dusk.

One time the mayor and I were scheduled to play on a Friday at Deepdale, a golf course on Long Island. He'd taped a radio show and asked me to meet him at the West 30th Street Heliport. When I got there, I met a gentleman I assumed was the pilot and asked him which seat I should sit in. I didn't want to take the mayor's seat. But he set me straight. "The mayor is the pilot," he said. I knew from the campaign that he was an avid helicopter pilot, but I had never flown with him before.

Mike flew us to Long Island and smoothly landed the helicopter. We played a great game, and then Mike asked me if I wanted a ride home. He meant literally—he was going to drop me off in Westchester County.

I thought, this is the most unbelievable experience of my life, flying around New York City with Mayor Bloomberg. It further strengthened my belief that golf was a great bonding system. Of course, we talked about politics, we talked about the future. But most important, we just had fun.

I learned a lot about leadership from playing with Mayor Mike. He told me:

1. If you make a promise, you keep a promise.

2. It's easier to say no than to say yes—and no idea is too big if it could make an impact.

3. Golf is more fun when you have something to do before and after. Golf can't be the only thing you do in a day.

14

GOLFERS-IN-CHIEF

Since I've spent a good portion of my professional career in the political world, no book of mine about golf would be complete without a nod to our presidential golfers. I believe it's very good for the nation when presidents play golf. All the positive aspects of the game—the relaxation, the stress reduction, the ability to focus on something inconsequential, being outdoors in nature, and the social bonding—can help a president in his job.

Golf has been a great presidential pastime ever since William Howard Taft wielded a club in the first decade of the twentieth century. President Taft was such an avid golfer that Theodore Roosevelt, who preceded him in the White House, warned him against playing. Roosevelt thought the elitist nature of the sport would lose Taft votes when he ran for reelection. Taft disputed the notion that golf was elitist. "I know that there is nothing more democratic than golf," he wrote. "There is nothing which furnishes a greater test of character and self-restraint, nothing which puts one more on an equality with one's fellows, or, I may say, puts one lower than one's fellows, than the game of golf."

Whether golf had anything to do with it, Taft lost the election in 1912 to Woodrow Wilson, but it turned out that Wilson was also quite the golfer. According to presidentialgolftracker.com, he played more than one thousand rounds of golf as president. He was so into the game that he painted his balls black so he could play in the snow.

As the twentieth century progressed and golf became more common, the interest was often reflected at the White House. Warren Harding, who died two years into his presidency, loved golf so much that he was on the course the day he was elected president. During his time in office, he enjoyed hitting balls on the White House lawn and had his dog, Laddie Boy, retrieve them. He loved the social aspects of golf, and for him it was all about having fun. It didn't matter that he wasn't a great player.

Franklin D. Roosevelt was an enthusiastic golfer and a star during his college years when he won the club championship at the family summer resort at Campobello Island Golf Club in New Brunswick, Canada. Tall, lean, and athletic, he was a natural. But after he contracted polio at the age of thirty-nine, he could no longer play. Eleanor Roosevelt once said of her husband, "The only thing that stands out as evidence of how he suffered when he finally knew that he would never walk again was the fact that I never heard him mention golf from the day he was taken ill. That game epitomized to him the ability to be out of doors and to enjoy the use of his body."

According to Michael Trostel, former curator of the USGA Museum and director of the World Golf Hall of Fame, FDR made an impact on golf that went beyond his ability to play the game, with a public works program that involved the construction of more than three hundred municipal golf courses. It was his way of making golf available to all.

Dwight "Ike" Eisenhower was one of the most prolific golfers to ever inhabit the White House. One of his favorite golf companions was Arnold Palmer. Ike installed a putting green on the South Lawn, and he wore his cleats in the Oval Office, so he could easily step out to hit balls—even though the cleats scarred the floor. Golf was his favorite way to relieve stress, although he would rage at the squirrels for interfering with his game. At one point he arranged to have the South Lawn squirrels captured and shipped off to Rock Creek Park.

As I described earlier, Eisenhower famously had a "little White House" known as Ike's Cabin installed at Augusta National Golf Club, where it remains to this day, filled with memorabilia.

Eisenhower's successor, John F. Kennedy, made Eisenhower's golf obsession a campaign issue in 1960, suggesting that the president's time at the golf course might better be spent on the people's business, and if elected Kennedy would be more attentive to the job. It was an unfair accusation, of course, and purely political in that it masked Kennedy's own enjoyment of the game. A story made the rounds that while in California for the campaign, Kennedy was playing golf one day at Cypress Point when his ball began rolling toward the par 3 sixteenth hole. He completely lost his composure, yelling, "No! No!" But when the ball didn't go in, he breathed a sigh of relief, knowing if word got out that he'd scored a hole in one, people would compare him to Eisenhower and say he was just another golfer trying to get into the White House. When he did reach the White House, however, JFK enjoyed playing at Burning Tree Golf Club in Washington, DC, and he was a pretty good golfer.

Lyndon Johnson was a transactional golfer. LBJ played the game as a way of corralling political allies. But he demanded proper obsequiousness, stating frankly, "One lesson you better learn if you want to be in politics is that you never go out on a golf course and beat the president."

Nixon wasn't a natural golfer. He only took up the game when he was in his forties, and never loved it. Like LBJ, he was more of a transactional player. His successor, Gerald Ford, was a true athlete, and he loved golf. However, he had a reputation for hitting spectators with his balls, which underscored the narrative that he was clumsy. The comedian Bob Hope once quipped, "It's not hard to find Jerry Ford on a golf course—you just follow the wounded." Ford was in on the joke, once telling an interviewer, "My game's getting better, and the best evidence is I'm hitting fewer spectators."

Ronald Reagan was a legendary member of Los Angeles Country Club, although he preferred horses. But George H. W. Bush was a passionate golfer. It was a family sport. Bush's grandfather had served as president of the USGA, and he and Barbara actually met at the Round Hill Club in Greenwich, Connecticut. He was eighteen and she was sixteen. Bush was involved with golf his entire life, in and out of the White House, and was a member of the World Golf Hall of Fame. He was respected for his prolific work with golf-related charities, including serving as honorary chairman of the First Tee, a youth development organization. He was also known for the speed of his game. The author James Patterson once played with him and reported: "It was a blur. The whole thing seemed to be a rush to get to the end. It was a feeling like, 'Wow, are we done now?'"

Bill Clinton is a dedicated golfer, and a very good golfer, notorious for redoing his shots—thus the term coined just for him, *billigans*. He's blatant about it. According to writer Rick Reilly who played with him in 1995 for a story, the Secret Service helped Clinton cheat, and it was all in good fun. Clinton relishes the social aspects of the game, and unlike his immediate predecessor, he'll stretch a game for as long as it lasts.

On February 15, 1995, Presidents Ford, Clinton, and George H. W. Bush played together at the Bob Hope Chrysler Classic at the Indian Wells Golf Club near Palm Springs, California. It was the first time three former presidents had golfed together, and a notably cordial reunion between the sitting president Clinton and Bush, the man he had defeated two years earlier. It was a wild scene. Both Ford and Bush hit spectators with balls, and one of Clinton's shots took out a piece of watermelon a young boy was eating. The event might have heralded the beginning of a close friendship between Bush and Clinton, which culminated in a joint mission to the earthquake devastated Haiti during the Obama administration.

Bush senior's son, George W., is a chip off the old block, also an avid golfer and contributor to golf-related causes, although as president he stopped playing in 2003 out of respect for the soldiers he had sent to war. He explained: "I don't want some mom whose son may have recently died to see the commander-in-chief playing golf. I feel I owe it to the families to be in solidarity as best as I can with them. And I think playing golf during a war just sends the wrong signal." His post-presidency has been his most successful period as a golfer. He made his first hole in one at Trinity Forest Golf Course in 2019 at the age of seventy-two.

Obama is serious about the game, and rigorously honest about following the rules. The CBS correspondent Mark Knoller, who keeps track of such things, reported that Obama spent about a thousand hours playing 214 rounds of golf as president, and yet not a great deal was known about his game because he tended to play privately. But someone who'd golfed with Obama told the *New York Times*, "If you came down from Mars and saw his disposition on the golf course, you would think he would be a pretty good president. He's honest, he keeps his composure through terrible adversity, he's unruffled, he smiles, and he doesn't quit."

It's always amusing that during election campaigns, candidates will inevitably accuse the other side of spending too much time on the golf course—the most recent example being Donald Trump, an inveterate golfer and owner of golf courses, accusing Obama of playing too much golf. Arguably no president has been as golf-immersed as Trump. His golf courses are among the best in the world, and he has uniquely demonstrated the power of golf for policy, diplomacy, and in relationships. Most presidential golfers have used the game as a break from the pressures of the job. Trump uses it to conduct presidential business. If the typical president wields the power of the Oval Office,

Trump wields that same power on the golf course, where he is in his element. The golf course is his domain, and when you see him golfing with senators like Lindsey Graham or world leaders, you know that business is being done.

Joe Biden has also been a strong golfer. During a presidential debate in July 2024, before he ended his campaign for a second term, Biden and Trump got into a tussle about their golf prowess. It was a pure testosterone-fueled standoff. Trump began by bragging: "I just won two club championships, not even senior, two regular club championships. To do that, you have to be quite smart, and you have to be able to hit the ball a long way. And I do it. He [Biden] doesn't do it. He can't hit a ball fifty yards. He challenged me to a golf match. He can't hit a ball fifty yards."

"I'd be happy to have a driving contest with him," Biden replied. "I got my handicap, when I was vice president, down to a six. And by the way, I told you before, I'm happy to play golf if you carry your own bag. Think you can do it?"

Trump scoffed. "That's the biggest lie, that he's a 6 handicap, of all."

Biden corrected. "I was 8 handicap."

"Yeah," Trump replied sarcastically. "I've seen your swing, I know your swing."

The golf-off never happened because Biden left the campaign weeks after the debate. But to paraphrase Trump, it would have been wild.

PRESIDENTS PLAYING: IT'S A GOOD THING

During a press conference while he was president, Eisenhower took a stab at explaining why taking a sports break was a healthy and productive choice. "There are three that I like all for the same reason, golf, fishing, and shooting, and I do because first, they take you into the fields. There is mild exercise, the kind that an older individual probably should have. And on top of it, it induces you to take at any one time two or three hours, if you can, where you are thinking of the bird or that ball or the wily trout. Now, to my mind, it is a very healthful, beneficial kind of thing, and I do it whenever I get a chance, as you well know."

Bill Clinton would agree. He told *Golf Digest* in 2020 that golf serves many positive purposes for him. He loves it, he said, because "it's a friendly game," and "I like it because it takes so much time." He explains:

"A lot of days like today, I'll come out here and I may go five holes before I get a good shot. But in the end, you can't do well if you're thinking about anything else. You can't play this game and think about anything else. And also, it's a place where—even though you've got these Secret Service people all around us—this is the nearest I ever am to being like a normal person. I'm alone playing with friends. It reminds me of everything I loved about my childhood and nature."

15

CHARACTER ON THE COURSE

Golf is a value-based sport. It's also a sport that self-regulates. You call the penalties on yourself. There is no referee on the course. You might get an opponent who will suggest that maybe there shouldn't be a penalty. But at the end of the day, it is up to the individual player to do the right thing.

In golf, if you get away with stuff, and you don't call it on yourself, that's called cheating. And who wants to play any sport or do any activity or be in business with someone who's a cheater? I've found that one of the things that attracts people to golf and makes them want to come back is your honesty and integrity. In most clubs, if you're cheating about the rules, or if you're moving the ball when you shouldn't or not calling a penalty, people won't want to play with you. It's as simple as that.

There are many ways to cheat at golf, including moving the ball and lying about the number of strokes.

There aren't many famous examples of pros cheating. It's certainly rare for high-stakes televised games. But one recent example involved Justin Doeden, playing the PGA Tour Canada in 2023. Doeden replaced the eighteenth hole double bogey with a par, and his competitors caught him in the act. He had to drop out of the tournament.

Later, Doeden issued an apology: "I am here to confess of the biggest mistake I have made in my life to date. I cheated in golf. This is not who I am. I let my sponsors down. I let my competitors down. I let my family down. I let myself down. I pray for your forgiveness."

Jerry Tarde, editor-in-chief of *Golf Digest,* put it well: "Rich or poor, low- or high-handicapper, the often-repeated consensus is that people who cheat in life don't necessarily cheat at golf, but people who cheat at golf invariably cheat in life."

Golf teaches you to take ownership— like calling penalties on yourself. If we can all learn to self-referee, it will be a better world for sure.

—EARL COOPER,
Eastside Golf

BEHAVE!

Character isn't just about whether or not you cheat on the golf course. "You learn about character on the golf course," Steve Gilbert offered. "Someone who throws his club, someone who is rude to caddies and staff. Someone who cheats, someone who is not thoughtful about the game or his partners—I won't do a deal with that person." I think most people feel the same way. A golf game serves as a microcosm of the rest of life, with highs and lows, success and disappointment. Your ability to meet the challenges and not be a jerk to your fellow golfers is indicative of how you behave in other situations.

JEFF SMITH—
Character Is King

Jeff Smith knows you can learn a lot about someone on the golf course. "Golf brings people together for a handful of hours," he said. "And they get to learn how they're going to react to situations socially and under pressure and how they react to things, and it makes them understand the person. As they observe and communicate, they're asking themselves, 'Do I want to do business with this person or not?' Because golf tends to expose character. You can't hide it through a round of golf."

Jeff calls golf a "value-based game, related to how you're valuing your time with another person." He has identified several signs of character that are clear during a game of golf.

INTEGRITY: Are you a person willing to bend or break the rules?

HANDLING STRESS: Golfers will put themselves under a lot of stress in front of people they barely know, or people they're trying to impress for one reason or another. Their reaction to the outcome of their golf shot tells you a lot over the course of a round of golf. You can see how someone handles the good and the bad.

GENEROSITY: Did you help me find my ball? Did you patiently wait for me? Were you happy when I made a good shot? There's an empathy and generosity inherent in golf. No one wants to root for a bad outcome for the other guy—even when you're competing. As a good golfer, you focus on your own game, not on rooting against someone. Remember, it's about relationships. You want to be able to talk to the person after the game.

Do I want to do business with this
person or not? Because golf tends
to expose character. You can't hide
it through a round of golf.

—JEFF SMITH

ANDY HARDIMAN—
The Fun of It

When I asked Andy Hardiman, instructor at Waccabuc Golf Club where he saw golf headed ten to fifteen years down the road, he had a fascinating answer—the nine-hole golf course. "We're concerned about climate change and water shortages," he said. "We're seeing that younger golfers don't necessarily want to play the long game. I see nine-hole courses opening up everywhere."

I think he was on to something. Already, the most popular form of golf is nine holes. Once that would have been viewed as a cop-out, but that's not true anymore. People happily play nine holes with their families and friends and they're not ashamed—they're having fun. I'm with Andy. I'd like to get the word out that it's okay to play nine holes—and in many cases it's even better.

Andy confirmed it. "At Waccabuc Country Club, if we look at where our increase in rounds is coming from, it's from people who are playing nine-hole events. Many times, these are families or friends outings. They plan a two-hour outing, play nine holes, and then have dinner.

The whole purpose of playing golf is fun. It gets us away from the stresses of life. Not a lot of people have four hours, but they can manage two hours to play nine holes."

Andy's main point was about having fun and being comfortable on the course. He certainly agrees with me about the importance of the deep relationships that get built on the golf course. And Andy and I have developed that kind of bond.

Andy inspires me with his joy and love of teaching. "I want to help people become better golfers so they can enjoy playing more. I like to welcome new players into the game and help them get situated into a social group. In many ways I'm a natural teacher. I think had I not been a golf pro, I might have been a high school algebra teacher."

It takes all kinds on a golf course, and Andy respects them all. "There's the guy that maybe has been playing for a very long time, and his idea of not embarrassing himself is being able to shoot in the low seventies. And then there's somebody who's totally brand new to it, whose score means nothing to them. They just want to be able to hit shots, advance the ball, and play a round without slowing everybody down.

"But this idea of being embarrassed. When you're playing out there, nobody is really watching you. Nobody's really concerned about your score, as long as you're a good person, you're good company, and you're fun to be around. That's more important than your score."

I agree with Andy on that point. I've observed the same thing for as long as I've played golf. That doesn't mean we're not all trying to improve in our own ways or aren't thrilled when we do well. Andy sees that side too. "We're all capable of hitting good shots," he said. "Maybe not consistently, but those moments are memorable for people. They're not going to remember their misses. They're going to remember the shot that they hit with the 7-iron from 120 yards on the third hole, and they hit it to ten feet. That's what they're going to remember—it's imprinted on the brain."

I could relate. After twenty-two years of lessons loving everything about golf, I wonder if golf will ever allow me to score better, and I'm not sure it even matters. But I sometimes feel like Don Quixote—in a comfortable way.

A GREAT FIRST DATE

Fore the Girls cofounder Cailyn Henderson told me the golf course is the perfect setting for a first date. "You can tell so much about someone from playing, even if it's only three holes. Golf exposes a lot. You can tell if they have anger issues, you can see how their etiquette is. You can tell if they know how to deal with failure—that's a big one. If I were to answer a question about what golf has taught me, it would be that it's taught me so much about how to deal with failure because in life—and in golf—you fail more times than you succeed. It teaches you how to pick yourself back up. And playing golf with someone exposes that ability in them."

I had to laugh a bit at the idea of going on a golfing first date with a golf pro. "I give that guy a lot of credit," I said to Cailyn.

Cofounder Margaret Wentz added, "My boyfriend and I both played golf—he played at DePauw. We went on a first date and we golfed nine holes, and we've been together ever since—four years. We knew right after the third hole that we were going to be together."

Of course, I wanted to know why, and Margaret obliged me. "He was super kind. He was out there to have fun. We talked a lot. There was great chemistry. He wasn't looking at his phone. He was fully present, and all those positive qualities came through on the course."

YOU'RE NEVER TOO YOUNG TO BUILD CHARACTER

I was excited to speak with Greg McLaughlin, the president and CEO of the PGA Tour First Tee Foundation. Greg has an impressive history in organized golf. He is the past president of PGA Tour Championships, former CEO of the Tiger Woods Foundation, and former vice president of business development for the BMW Championship. His current position with First Tee is all about an endeavor near and dear to my heart—bringing kids into the game. Having just celebrated its twentieth year, First Tee has seen an astounding 15 million kids come through its program. These kids represent a wide range of backgrounds. "The scope is enormous," Greg told me. "It's about as inclusive as any organization can be. I think we boast the most successful reach in golf in all aspects, including reaching underserved communities and being gender diverse."

The kids are great—willing to learn and engage with one another. "Kids are more social by nature," Greg said. "And some of the kids come mostly for socialization. But the core idea is that golf is a strong platform to make that introduction. They meet kids from all fifty states, and if they come to our Game Changers Academy or our Leadership Academy, they learn not only skills but are in an environment where they can develop strong character."

Greg emphasized, "Golf requires a level of honesty and integrity. It's just inherent in the game, and you hear people talk about how, at the professional level, or even at the amateur level, that individuals will disqualify themselves because they inadvertently violated a rule, and they turn themselves in. There's not any other sport that has that, and the First Tee is the beginning of it. It was founded and built on core values. And they're an element of the curriculum, which goes beyond what's inherent in the game. And it's very intentional about life skills, which is integrated into our golf curriculum. That's what our program is built on. You can learn life skills through the game."

Our daughter, Isabella, goes in and out of golf. She has the most beautiful swing; she played for her high school golf team, but she does not share the passion that Marcela, Matthew, and I have. In some ways, it's a shame because she has a wonderful natural ability. On the other hand, I get it. Golf is a lot. A lot of clubs, keeping track of a lot of numbers, dress codes, tee times. Shots that don't go where you want.

When Isa was on the Hackley golf team in high school, she told me about a match she was playing against the Riverdale team, and her opponent had counted a different number of strokes for a hole than Isa did. Golf is an honor sport; your stroke count is your stroke count, but if you disagree with your opponent there is no replay monitor or referee. You just move on. It can get exhausting and quite frankly discouraging to get into petty disagreements on each hole.

For me, that is where the civility of golf comes into play. Golf is a self-refereed sport. Your word is your honor. You either play by the rules, count your strokes, or I doubt I am playing with you again. Isa felt the same way that day at Sleepy Hollow.

SHAWN LINDO—
It's Just a Game

Shawn Lindo is a professional bodybuilder with twenty-plus years of experience and owner of skylevelfitness since 2009. In addition, he's a personal trainer, mentor, and motivational speaker, and incidentally has also been an extra on several TV shows and movies. He is also the CEO of Black Muscle Golf, an online golf apparel company that caters to fit, muscular golfers.

In my book, Shawn is also an amateur philosopher.

"Golf is very similar to regular life," he told me. "You can have fun in regular life. You can hang out with your friends, go to a bar, go out for dinner. And there are going to be challenges that happen as well. How you deal with those, and how you support each other as friends can make a huge difference.

"Golf is like that too. The same principles apply. You might be on the golf course, having a lousy couple of holes, or worse. How do you respond? Are you throwing your clubs and cursing? Are you angry? Are you taking it out on your friends?

"I stay cool when I play, and people ask me, 'How do you not let it get to you?' I ask, 'Why should I let it get to me? At the end of the day, we're playing a game. We're not professionals.' And we're not professionals at life, either. We're going through it and learning how to handle it as we go."

PART 4

MASTERING
THE GAME

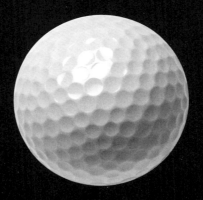

16

PLAY GOLF AND GET FIT

When I speak to golfers, they often talk about how they get a "two-fer." They get to play a sport that they love, and they get to achieve an exercise goal for the day. Most golf courses require six miles of walking if you're playing eighteen holes. If you're carrying your golf bag, all the better. We can also assume that golfers will take 150 to 200 swings, including practice swings, while they're playing. All of these activities factor into the fitness profile of golf. Most golfers care about this to some extent and want to know how golf fits into overall health: weight loss, strength training, cardiovascular fitness, mobility, and flexibility.

Golf is not always given its due as an optimal sport for fitness. Reflecting on his journey to embrace golf, my friend Steve Gilbert recalled, "I not only did not play golf, but I disdained people who played golf because I thought it was non-aerobic. For all the years I ran all my private equity companies, if people played golf, I kind of looked down on them a little bit because I didn't really understand it." Steve enjoyed a variety of highly aerobic sports like squash and basketball. "It just never dawned on me when I was forty-five or fifty that I'd have artificial knees one day and would have to rethink fitness."

GALE BERNHARDT—
The Fitness Benefits of Golf

One would think that an outing on a golf course would be a good source of fitness, especially if you walk the course. However, like Steve, many exercise buffs look down on it as a lackluster exercise opportunity. I turned to Gale Bernhardt, a leading athletic trainer and two-time Olympic coach, for advice. I've known Gale for many years, and she collaborated with me on my 2015 book *Become a Fat-Burning Machine*. I asked Gale to describe the health benefits of golfing.

She gave me an overview—kind of a formula. You start golfing by going to the driving range and practicing a couple times per week. Golf and overall fitness are improved because of training principles: People are consistent (frequency), they progress to more holes (duration), they can move about the course faster (intensity), they end up golfing more (frequency × duration = volume). In order to improve without injury, they need to carefully increase the amount of golf they do (progressive overload) and be sure to include rest and recovery.

Gale agreed that golf is a great form of exercise, offering several health benefits—although she underlines that golfers should walk as often as possible. That's not to say golfing is a complete exercise. While you might benefit from walking on the golf course, you should supplement it with other activities. Here's Gale's analysis.

BENEFITS OF WALKING THE GOLF COURSE

Cardiovascular Health: Walking is a great cardiovascular exercise. It increases heart rate and blood flow, contributing to overall heart and lung health. An eighteen-hole course could yield 10,000 to 13,000 steps.

Calorie Burning: Walking eighteen holes can cover a distance of four to six miles, helping burn a significant number of calories—up to 2,000—which is beneficial for weight management.

Muscle Endurance: The activity requires endurance, particularly in the legs, as golfers traverse various terrains over several hours.

Mental Health: Walking can reduce stress and anxiety, improve mood, and enhance mental well-being. Walking increases the production of endorphins, releases serotonin and norepinephrine, which help with depression, anxiety, and stress relief.

LIMITATIONS AND WHY
THE PROGRESS MAY BE SHORT-LIVED

Lack of Movement Diversity: Golf course walking is primarily based on steady-state cardio combined with some rapid bursts (ball striking). As you already know, golf and our daily life activities require our body to move in different planes of motion. In addition, as we get older, we lose muscle size, strength, balance, and range of motion. A well-rounded fitness program should be added to walking the course to achieve a better fitness level.

Specific Strength and Flexibility Needs: Golfers who want to improve their golf game or want their body to handle the stress from the golf swing require specific strength, mobility, and rotational power to improve, which walking doesn't adequately provide.

Risk of Overuse Injuries: Repeatedly walking the same courses without varied exercise can lead to overuse injuries due to the lack of muscular balance and strength training. Additionally, those who have the time to golf multiple times per day and week risk overuse injuries. These injuries can force you to take time away from golf, which no one wants.

Insufficient Intensity for Advanced Fitness Goals: For those with higher fitness aspirations, like professional golfers or athletes, walking a golf course doesn't meet the intensity required for advanced conditioning.

Adaptation and Plateauing: The body is remarkably adaptable. As you regularly walk, your body becomes more efficient. This efficiency means that over time, the same distance and pace of walking will provide less of a cardiovascular challenge.

Diminishing Returns: As your cardiovascular system adapts to the demands of walking, the rate of improvement in your cardiovascular fitness will slow down, and eventually, you may hit a plateau.

Limited Intensity: Walking is generally a low to moderate-intensity exercise. To significantly improve cardiovascular fitness, especially for those who are already somewhat fit, higher-intensity exercises are often necessary.

While walking the golf course is beneficial and a good form of exercise, especially for those who are otherwise sedentary, it's important for golfers to engage in a more comprehensive fitness program. This program should include mobility training, stability training, resistance training, power training, and heart rate-based endurance training.

The solution to the shortcomings is to focus on overall fitness as a way of improving your golf performance and your health goals. For that I turned to Loic Descoutures.

LOIC DESCOUTURES—
Training for Golf Excellence

While basic fitness goals might work fine for many people, some are interested in a more challenging fitness goal that can be achieved as well. I talked with Loic Descoutures, the CEO of Train 2 Excel in Ridgefield, Connecticut, which offers a golf lab and training program.

There are three parts to the program:

1. Identifying the foundation of your swing: A thorough assessment will help you understand where your current body swing connection is and how to improve it.

2. Improving movement and increasing the distance of your drive: A program to help you become a more efficient golfer through a customized training plan.

3. Helping you move better, increase efficiency, and prevent injury: A program of continuous improvement in your mobility, stability, strength, and speed, so you can reach new goals in your game and remain injury-free.

Loic is part of a new trend to incorporate fitness goals with golf. "Before the 1990s, the focus of golf professionals was predominantly on selecting the right equipment, enhancing their mental game, and perfecting their golf swing," he explained to me. "However, in the mid-1990s, Tiger Woods revolutionized golf conditioning, changing the way professionals approached their training. Now, the modern approach to golf training encompasses not only instruction, equipment, and the mental aspect of the game but also physical conditioning.

"The demands of the golf swing require the golfer to stabilize the body, rotate effectively, and generate power in a repetitive manner. Professional golfers utilize high-end technology to analyze their swing and make biomechanical improvements. Additionally, they engage in physical screenings to understand how their body's movement affects their swing. For professional golfers, gym sessions are considered as crucial as practicing swings at the driving range. They focus on improving specific physical qualities essential for enhancing their swing or maintaining the abilities that enable them to perform at their best.

"The philosophy underlying this training regimen is known as the joint-by-joint approach, as defined by Mike Boyle and Gray Cook. This approach suggests that the body is a series of interdependent segments requiring either mobility or stability. A deficiency in one area can lead to compensatory movements in another, potentially leading to inefficiency and injury."

What should a training session look like?

Loic designed a general training recommendation for this book, based on those fitness goals. He recommends that the initial step in any training session involves five minutes of steady-paced cardio to increase body temperature, followed by a soft tissue segment using a foam roller. Foam rolling benefits include improved muscle elasticity and improved movement quality.

Following this, the mobility segment begins, targeting the ankles, hips, thoracic spine, and shoulder girdle.

Once mobility is improved, it's necessary to increase stability, as defined by the Titleist Performance Institute, which ensures efficient energy transfer and reduces the risk of injury during the swing. In this section we will target especially the hips, lumbar spine, and shoulders.

With the body now better prepared, the next phase involves a dynamic warm-up, rehearsing movement patterns that will be used in subsequent sections of the training.

Next is the power section focusing on both the upper and lower body through exercises like speed work, medicine ball throws, plyometrics, and, in some cases, Olympic lifting.

Next we have our strength training segment. Strength training does not isolate muscles but rather focuses on movement patterns such as the hinge, squat, push, pull, and rotation that are crucial for golf.

It's important to note that logical exercise progression tailored to individual goals is crucial for achieving desired results. Muscle groups require at least six to eight sessions to achieve maximal outcomes, indicating that changing exercises every gym visit is not advisable.

A practical way to start is with a two-day program, providing a structured approach to enhance golf performance through physical conditioning.

Here is an example of a training session designed to help you move better, play better, and reduce your risk of injuries:

GOLF CONDITIONING TRAINING SESSION

For more specific instructions, please go to train2xcel.com and click on their golf fitness page.

CARDIO: 5 MIN

SOFT TISSUE: 1 X 30 SEC EACH

Calves

Hamstrings

Glutes

Upper Back

Lats

Outer Thigh

Quads/Hip Flexors

Adductors

MOBILITY

Leg Lowering

Sidelying T Spine Rotation

Bretzel 2

Supine Glute Stretch

½ Kneeling Hip Flexor Stretch with Side Bend

½ Kneeling Open Stance Ankle Mobility

STABILITY

Plank on Knees

Plank

Bird Dog—1 Arm Reach Opposite Shoulder

Bird Dog—1 Arm Extension

½ Kneeling Torso Rotation with Dowel Hip Bridge

DYNAMIC WARM-UP

Bent Over T's

Miniband Side Walk

Standing Knee to Chest

Reverse Lunges with Torso Rotation

Standing Leg Cradle

Lateral Squat

Skipping in Place

POWER

Snap Down

Box Jump—No Counter Movement

½ Kneeling MB Chest Pass

STRENGTH

Assisted Bodyweight Squat

Goblet Squat

½ Kneeling Single Arm Low Angle Pulldown

RDL Knees Against Bench

2 DB Single Leg RDL—Kickstand

½ Kneeling Single Arm Cable Chest Press

CARDIO: 5 MIN

SOFT TISSUE: 1 X 30 SEC EACH

    Calves

    Hamstrings

    Glutes

    Upper Back

    Lats

    Outer Thigh

    Quads/Hip Flexors

    Adductors

MOBILITY (EXAMPLES)

    Leg Lowering

    Sidelying T Spine Rotation

    Bretzel 2

    Supine Glute Stretch

    ½ Kneeling Hip Flexor Stretch with Side Bend

    ½ Kneeling Open Stance Ankle Mobility

STABILITY (EXAMPLES)

    Side Plank on Knees

    Supine Pelvic Tilt

    ½ Kneeling Torso Rotation with Dowel

DYNAMIC WARM-UP (EXAMPLE)

    Bent Over T's

    Miniband Side Walk

Standing Knee to Chest

Reverse Lunges with Torso Rotation

Standing Leg Cradle

Lateral Squat

Skipping in Place

POWER

½ Kneeling MB Front Twist Throw

½ Kneeling MB Slams

STRENGTH

Toe Touch Progression

1 KB Sumo Deadlift

Elevated Push-Up

Push-Up

Rack Assisted Bodyweight Split Squat

Goblet Split Squat

½ Kneeling Single Arm Cable Row

17

BE IN THE MOMENT

It was summer 2022, and I was walking up the fifth fairway at one of my favorite golf courses in Aspen, Colorado. As I walked, I gazed at the incredible scenery, captivated by the pristine skies above Buttermilk Mountain, and the breathtaking setting. I couldn't help being filled with the moment—feeling my great fortune at being in Aspen among wonderful people. I'd been experiencing that same sense of wonder and gratitude for fifteen years.

This time I was a guest of my friend Tony at a tournament, along with others I've met at previous tournaments. Yet while I was pinching myself for being there, I was also painfully aware that I was playing so badly that I might never get invited back. I was shaking in my boots, because the game I love so much seemed to be leaving me. I'd lost my golf swing.

True, I had some big distractions going on. I was in the middle of the biggest business deal of my career. I'd built a company, for which I had a strong vision, after starting it in 2016 in the living room of my apartment in New York City, which happened to be undergoing renovation. I had seen the future of social media. I'd understood how momentum works and wrote a book about it called *Maximum Momentum.* I had wonderful people working for me, and a solid partner who had helped me build this incredible company. Now we were about to close the deal to sell the company, and my mind was so focused on the deal that I couldn't think of anything else.

In the process, my golf game had suffered what felt like a fatal blow. My timing was gone, my swing was gone, and I was incredibly sad and disappointed that this had happened to me.

As I looked around the amazing golf club in Aspen, where I had experienced such joy, I knew I might never return.

I was staying with Tony, and back at his house I was lamenting the fact that I'd lost my game, and I had to find someone to help me get it back. I couldn't bear the thought of giving up.

Tony's wife, Shelly, said, "It doesn't sound like you need another golf pro or a golf lesson. It sounds like you need a golf psychiatrist."

I looked at her and a light went on. "Oh, my God," I said. "You're right. I need a golf psychiatrist." And from that moment, I was committed to finding one.

I finished my business deal at the end of September, and I was staying in Vail. I began looking for someone to pull me through my block. I was lucky—there were performance coaches everywhere, because skiers can lose their way and need to refocus.

I found a psychiatrist, and the first thing he said was, "Tell me why you're here."

"I'm here because I've lost something that I love," I said. "I've lost my ability to golf."

He nodded, without quite getting it. "Okay . . ."

"I love golf," I explained, a little desperate. "And I can't do it. I can't swing the club. The ball goes crazy places. I want to get my swing back."

He was nodding, and I could see the wheels turning. I wondered if this had been such a great idea. Finally, he said: "Let's get some history. Think about the times you've done well."

Okay, I could do that. I told him about running three Ironman Triathlons in Kona, Hawaii, my most impressive physical achievement. I told him about losing seventy-five pounds and writing a diet book. I told him about working for several successful politicians. I told him about the work I did for big corporations. I told him about my thirty-plus years of marriage and my wonderful children.

"It sounds like you've been able to achieve a lot," he said. "What's wrong with your golf?"

I tried to explain. "I look at the ball," I said. "And I see it going . . ."

"You see the future?" he interjected.

"Yes." Needless to say, the future of the ball's trajectory didn't look great.

Then he asked, "When you go into a meeting, do you ever look ahead and think about people's negative reactions?"

"No."

"When you're training to run Ironman, do you imagine yourself tripping or falling off your bike or drowning?"

"No."

"But when you're golfing, you imagine the ball going in the woods or in the sand trap?"

"Yes." I was beginning to see where he was going.

"It sounds like you're seeing things that haven't happened yet," he noted. "You're seeing outcomes. You're seeing the ball go in the water. You're seeing the ball go out of bounds. In golf, you've got to really be in the moment. You can't go to the future and see what's going to happen. Because it'll play with your mind."

And then he gave me a drill that changed my life and my game. It works in every situation, including golf.

"Before you hit the ball, I want you to tell me five things you can see," he said. "Tell me four things you can hear. Tell me three things you can touch. Tell me two things you can smell. And after you do that, hit the ball."

We practiced right there in his office. "I see your computer, I see this chair, I see a door, I see a light, I see you." Then, "I hear us talking, I hear the fan, I hear voices in another room, I hear a phone ringing." Then, "The room smells a little musty, I can smell my sweat, I can smell food cooking." Then, "I can touch the chair, I can touch the doorknob." Then, "I can taste the gum I'm chewing."

He smiled. "How does that make you feel?"

"Focused," I said. "Grounded."

"Good. Now apply that to your golf game. You already know how to be in the moment in many situations, but with golf, other thoughts are coming into your head that interrupt the flow of you and the ball. Picture a leaf floating down a stream. You can't let the leaf get caught up. You have to keep the flow going."

I left his office and before I played golf the next time, I went skiing. And I applied the lesson of being in the moment. I am a pretty good skier. I'm aggressive, but I'm always a little hesitant. I got to the top of the mountain, and I let it flow. I skied like I'd never skied before in my life. I realized it was because I wasn't thinking about falling. The skis were moving, and I was going with them. It was a revelation.

A few days later, I was on the golf course, getting ready to play, and I put myself through the mental exercise, teasing each one of my senses, fully inhabiting my body in the moment on this glorious course. And when I was ready, I swung. The club moved smoothly, and the ball sailed into the air, hurling in the right direction. The sun shone down on the green, and I knew I was back.

18

TOP OF THE PEGBOARD

Since I started golfing, Pine Valley has always been the top ranked course on the *Golf Digest* pegboard, which you'll remember is my aspirational list of the one hundred greatest courses. I could tell you it was my aspiration to play at Pine Valley one day, but that would be a lie. I had never expected to play Pine Valley. Not that it was so hard to get to. I live in New York, and Pine Valley is in Southwest Jersey, near Philadelphia. An easy trip down I-95.

The reason I never expected to play Pine Valley is its reputation for being one of the toughest courses in the world. In 2023, in a separate ranking, *Golf Digest* chose the most challenging courses, and Pine Valley came out on top there as well—"forged from the sandy pine barrens . . . [blending] all three schools of golf design—penal, heroic, and strategic—often times on a single hole." Terrifying!

I'd read up on Pine Valley, not to torment myself, but to confirm my opinion. I learned about how the course design philosophy is based on penal architecture and required the use of every club in the bag. Each hole is so specific that it would be the signature hole at any other golf course. Frankly, I didn't think I was good enough to play there, so I never bothered to try.

And then as I was working on this book, my attitude started to change. I realized that playing Pine Valley would be the pinnacle of my aspiration to be a golfer who could actually play the number one course in the world with some skill. So, in the summer of 2024, I set out to play Pine Valley. Fortunately, William and Jay knew a member—Michael Bamberger. Michael and William had been friends in college. He also happened to be one of the most famous and prolific golf writers around. His classic *To the Linksland* is still considered one of the great books of all time about golf and self-discovery, thirty years after he wrote it. Michael has written other golf books, and he writes regularly for golf magazines. He's the kind of person I instantly find interesting.

I'd met Michael briefly when I played in the American Express tournament in Palm Springs in January. He was undercover giving out swag—working on his next project. I knew I recognized him and after a few minutes of staring at each other, I introduced myself and mentioned that we had friends in common—William and Jay. I later found that we actually had many more. We chatted for a while; the kind of golf networking people do. It was all very friendly.

When Jay arranged with Michael to have a foursome with me and William on Labor Day weekend at Pine Valley, I thought it might become the most significant golf adventure of my life. I always love playing with my buddies—as you know by now. And having Michael there as the member who guided us, as our Sherpa, and being so knowledgeable about golf, made it much more special. I knew going in that it would be an unforgettable experience.

We arrived at Pine Valley and had lunch before playing. I noted the atmosphere of the place that had always intimidated me. It was very low-key and subtle. I relaxed somewhat over lunch, but I was still nervous as we walked out onto the course. I imagined that Greg was there with me, looking down and watching me play Pine Valley.

On the first hole on the tee box, there's a small sign, "No mulligans." In other words, no takebacks. You hit your shot and then you go play it. That spoke to me because my life motto could be "No mulligans."

Michael suddenly said, "Oh, I forgot to give you a scorecard." And then he smiled. "Well, this isn't a USGA-sanctioned game. I don't think we need to keep score." I looked at him in disbelief and delight. This was all I ever wanted, to go out and play for the sheer pleasure of it without having to keep score. We would play without counting shots or worrying about birdies or mulligans. It would just be golf with friends at Pine Valley.

So, I went up to the tee box at Pine Valley, the number one golf course in the world, and I hit a mediocre tee shot. *Uh-oh, what kind of day would this be?* And then I ripped the most perfect 175-yard approach shot that landed right in front of the green. High, long, swoosh—the most perfect sound of golf as the ball left my club.

As we walked along to the first green, Michael said, "Look at this rough." I looked down and noticed that it wasn't the pristine grass I was used to from other courses—brown, sandy, a little longer than the fairway but not by much. This rough was *really* rough. "We don't need that tall, thick grass that's overly green," Michael said. "This is what rough looks like. Rough is scruff." I quickly wrote that down on the scorecard that I had tucked in my back pocket. We weren't keeping score, but I was definitely taking notes.

I soon realized why Pine Valley is the number one golf course in the country. Each hole is distinctive and uniquely challenges your strategy, competency, and ability to think two or three shots ahead. Each hole is carved out of the earth, as if it appeared that way naturally through evolution. There are no bunkers, just waste areas. I'd brought twenty-four balls because I expected to lose a lot of them. But I only lost one ball. You don't lose your ball—that would be too easy—you have to play them all. Much more challenging!

The difficulty of the course gave our group more time to play and to talk. Without a score, the pressure was off. We admired one another's shots. We knew when we got a par, we knew when we got a birdie (Michael had two!), and I suspect we knew when we didn't finish the hole, or at least I knew when I didn't finish a hole, and I wasn't ashamed. Throughout this book I've been talking about my dream game: an excuse for four friends to walk around in a gorgeous setting and have a great time together. This was it, with the added thrill that it was happening at Pine Valley.

As we were approaching the final holes, I noticed that Michael was making some putts lefty and others righty. He was making birdies both ways. I thought it was unusual, and I wondered if it was a technique I was unfamiliar with. So, I asked him.

Michael told me he had the yips, and that was the reason. The yips are wrist spasms that come on during putting. They definitely happen as we get older, although there's some evidence that golfers of all ages get the yips. Tiger Woods has even confessed that it has happened to him.

I was surprised to hear that Michael had the yips, because he'd been putting well all day. On the eighteenth hole, he had an eight- to ten-foot putt. I was standing close to him, and he said, "I feel a yip coming on. Would you take this putt for me?" It was a super straight uphill putt. As straightforward as they get at Pine Valley. An overwhelming warmth went through my body, my mind went calm. I was on the putting green with Michael Bamberger's putter in my hand.

Let me underscore the point that this was incredibly unusual. You don't give someone else your putter. You have to make your own shots. But I understood that Michael was doing something much more symbolic. He was asking me to make the last putt of the day at Pine Valley. I felt the electricity of holding his putter, lined it up, and missed it by a few inches.

It didn't matter. Standing there I felt the power of golf. The power of the friendliness of golf. The social power. The thrill of having someone ask me to putt their last putt using their putter.

Michael is a golf writer who appreciates the meaning of such moments. Whether he had the yips or not, he knew what he was doing. It was like the legendary broadcaster Walter Cronkite giving me the mic and letting me perform his famous sign-off for his news broadcast.

The last putt of the day. The sign-off: "And that's the way it is on September 2, 2024, at Pine Valley."

TOMORROW IS A NEW DAY

Over the period that I was working on this project, my relationship with golf changed. I started living some of the principles of this book, such as playing nine is fine. I should practice a little more to start getting better. I stuck with the same golf clubs all year and was less of a gear head.

I have become more aware of why people golf. In a world that has become digital, golf is IRL whether you play on green grass or in a simulator. It is social—it involves human interactions. Golf can cross gender, race, social class, and age. It is full of shared experiences that bring people together.

Golf is emotional. It opens the mind to feelings. It makes you vulnerable. In most sports, you can experience feelings, but you don't have to. In golf, there is no choice. It is you and the ball. The ball is an inanimate object with no feelings. You are a person full of feelings. To make anything happen—stroke a putt, hit a drive, and so on. You need to do something, and you will have a reaction.

Golf is full of hope and optimism. No matter how well or how badly you play, you can't wait to play again. Golf leaves you with the belief that things will be better tomorrow. That tomorrow will be better than today. You can always get better.

The real opponent in golf is you. You are for and against yourself. No two shots are ever the same. And that's why you can't wait to find out what happens next.

MIKE'S TOP 50 GOLF COURSES

When I started golfing in the early nineties, I used *Golf Digest*'s America's 100 Greatest Golf Courses list to identify which courses were the highest ranked in the United States. I kept track of the courses I had played. As I started to travel more internationally, I expanded my reach and began using the World's 100 Greatest Courses list.

After thirty years playing golf, involving thousands of rounds, hundreds of tournaments, and countless lessons, I created my personal list of Top 50 Golf Clubs using my own "Dirty Dozen of Criteria."

Mike's Top 50 Golf Clubs is very specific to the type of golf experiences I have shared in the book. Here's my "Dirty Dozen of Criteria":

1. **Firsthand Knowledge:** Have I played the course?

2. **Fun:** Did I have fun with my friends and family?

3. **Design and Layout:** Were the holes interesting and different? Does it suit my game?

4. **Aesthetics and Scenery:** Did I gasp at the stunning views and beautiful landscape?

5. **Historical and Cultural Significance:** Is there a strong sense of tradition and tie to golf heritage?

6. **Condition:** Was the course in great shape?

7. **Quality of the Food:** Did I have good tasting healthy choices to eat?

8. **Play Again:** As soon as I finished, did I want to play the course again?

9. **Feel at Home There:** Do I know the fairways and the greens?

10. **Walkable:** Does the course have the option to walk it?

11. **Welcoming and Knowledgeable Staff and Pros:** Were they friendly and helpful at the club?

12. **Weather:** Is it typically nice weather—not rain, wind, or cold?

MY TOP 50

1. Augusta National Golf Club, Augusta, GA
2. Pine Valley Golf Club, Pine Valley, NJ
3. Cypress Point Club, Pebble Beach, CA
4. Los Angeles Country Club: North, Los Angeles, CA
5. Friar's Head Golf Club, Riverhead, NY
6. Eagle Springs Golf Club, Wolcott, CO
7. GlenArbor Golf Club, Bedford Hills, NY
8. Jockey Club Golf, Buenos Aires, Argentina
9. Waccabuc Country Club, Waccabuc, NY
10. Maroon Creek Club, Aspen, CO
11. La Barra Golf Club, Punta del Este, Uruguay
12. Quaker Ridge Golf Club, Scarsdale, NY
13. Öviinbyrd Golf Club, Muskoka, Canada

• ACKNOWLEDGMENTS •

As I have emphasized throughout this book, golf is a game of relationships, and I have been blessed with a great many people in my life—with the added bonus that they also join me on the golf course. First and foremost, my wife, Marcela, a tremendous golfer and constant inspiration, and my children, Matthew and Isabella. It's a joy to share their lives in every way, and a real treat to golf with them. A special mention of my late stepfather, Greg, who introduced me to golf and was my first golf buddy and mentor. I miss Greg. I miss my golf buddy.

Golf wouldn't be the same to me without my reliable buddies, who have been with me for my most memorable golfing adventures—William, Tony, Joe, Jim, Steve, Polly, Mark, Billy, Nat, Dick, and Sam, I love you guys.

There have also been significant instructors in my golf journey—David Gagnon, John McPhee, Andy Hardiman, Martin Granda, Max Rohrdan, and Jeff Smith. Each year I wanted to try something new, each year you listened, were patient, and brought me along. Malcolm Gladwell was right: It takes ten thousand hours to achieve true expertise. I wonder where I'm at.

Mike Bloomberg was an important influence on my professional life in many ways. He was an incredibly hard worker, and he showed me how golf could fit into a 24/7 lifestyle. My favorite Bloomberg quote was when Mike told me that golf was only fun if you had something to do before golf and after golf. It couldn't be the only activity of the day. There have been no truer words to live by. Everything is better with golf, but golf can't be all there is.

I am grateful to those who participated in interviews to help give this book breadth and depth. Your input and expertise have been invaluable contributions. Many thanks to Earl Cooper, Loic Descoutures, Debbie Doniger, Klaus Eldrup-Jørgensen, Gale Bernhardt, Shelli Bettman, David Gagnon, Ronan Galvin, Steve Gilbert, Martin Granda, Jay Haas, Cailyn Henderson, Haeshin Lee, Shawn Lindo, Stephen and Erica Malbon, Greg McLaughlin, Greg and Monica Pattison, Don Placek, Kenyatta Ramsey, Igor Reyes, Jason Richards, Jeff Smith, Jimmy Spencer, Artie Starrs, Jared Solomon, Keith Ward, and Margaret Wentz.

Deepest thanks to my publisher, Judith Regan, who always gets my vision and helps me make it sing. Judith's talent, insight, and enthusiasm have given this project the momentum to soar. I only have to say one sentence and Judith knows—and tells me to write it. She has her finger on the pulse of culture, and she knows what's next.

For a third time, the writer Catherine Whitney has been my partner in crime on this project. Catherine and I speak the same language and understand each other's thinking. She fully embraced the idea that golf can change your life, and our collaboration has been an exciting journey. I promised Catherine she would be a golfer by the time this book was published. I am putting it here in writing. Hopefully, we are reading this on the nineteenth hole at one of my favorite golf courses in Westchester.

And then there is Britt Kahn. This is our second book together—fifteen years apart! Britt believed in the power of golf from the first time we discussed this book. Britt knows everyone, everywhere, and was behind the scenes making the connections that helped elevate this book to a level of importance in the golf world. Her hard, smart work really paid off.

ACKNOWLEDGMENTS

Thanks too to Nancy Laracuenta who seamlessly coordinated the interviews and transcripts and never missed a beat. Finally, I want to acknowledge Alex Gibani, who rose to the occasion as an intern and official representative of Gen Z, proving the point that golf is for everybody.

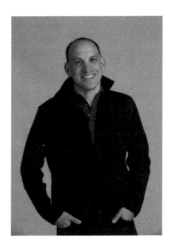

Best-selling author MIKE BERLAND is a strategic advisor and communications consultant with over thirty years of experience in consumer behavior and trends. MSNBC named him "The Genius Pollster."

Known for his political and business insight, he has appeared throughout the media, including on Fox Business Network's *Mornings with Maria*. He has also partnered with leading brands including Airbnb, OpenAI, Crocs, Estée Lauder Companies, StockX, Microsoft, Meta, and the National Hockey League.

His book *Not About Golf: About You and Golf* is a handbook for the golf-curious. Mike debunks the myths and stereotypes of golf while explaining how the momentum of golf creates social and networking benefits for everyone.

Mike is currently a senior partner at Penta Group. Previously, he was CEO of Edelman Berland and president of Penn, Schoen & Berland. He has served as chair of the Gotham Chapter of New York City's Young Presidents' Organization (YPO) and is a Commonwealth Scholar from the University of Massachusetts.

He is the author of *Maximum Momentum* and the national bestseller *Become a Fat-Burning Machine*.

An avid golfer, Mike enjoys playing courses worldwide, building connections, and rediscovering the joy of playing the game.